THE MAGIC OF HYDROGEN PEROXIDE

By Emily Thacker

Published by:

James Direct Inc

500 S. Prospect Ave.

Hartville, Ohio 44632

U.S.A.

This book is intended as a record of folklore and historical solutions and is composed of tips, suggestions, and remedies. It is sold with the understanding that the publisher is not engaged in rendering medical advice and does not intend this as a substitute for medical care by qualified professionals. No claims are intended as to the safety, or endorsing the effectiveness, of any of the remedies which have been included and the publisher cannot guarantee the accuracy or usefulness of individual remedies in this collection.

If you have a medical problem you should consult a physician.

ISBN: 978-1-62397-055-0

Printing 12 11 10 9 8 7 6 5 4 3

Seventh Edition   **Copyright 2010**   **James Direct Inc**

Books by Emily Thacker

The Vinegar Book

The Vinegar Book II

Vinegar and Tea

Vinegar Home Guide

The Vinegar Anniversary Book

Emergency Disaster Preparedness

Garlic: Nature's Natural Companion

The Magic of Baking Soda

The Magic of Hydrogen Peroxide

Eternal Youth: Turning Back the Hands of Time

The Honey Book

The Cinnamon Book

The Vinegar Formula Guide

The Hydrogen Peroxide Formula Guide

http://www.jamesdirect.com

Table of Contents

A Letter from Emily 5

Introduction. 11

Chapter One
Hydrogen Peroxide's Fascinating History 19

Chapter Two
Getting Started 51

Chapter Three
Hydrogen Peroxide and Better Health. 57

Chapter Four
Beauty, Skin Deep. 85

Chapter Five
Around the Home. 95

Chapter Six
The Great Outdoors 125

Chapter Seven
Foaming Fun 141

Chapter Eight
Emily Answers Your Questions About Hydrogen
        Peroxide. 153

Chapter Nine
A Word of Caution 161

Chapter Ten
Appendices 165

Index. 182

A Letter from Emily

Dear Reader,

It is a joy to come to you again with another wonderful collection of old-time home remedies. I cannot begin to tell you how many kind readers have written to me, asking when the sequel to *THE VINEGAR HOME GUIDE* would appear. Thank you! Your letters have been a real source of encouragement! Many of you have also shared your remembrances, and commented on the cleaning tips and new ideas you personally found to be the most useful.

One theme keeps reoccurring in your letters. Readers, from all across the world, relate how they have found hydrogen peroxide to be a part of better health and easier cleaning. As I read your letters, I see a continuing concern for maintaining good health without a lot of prescription drugs and doctor visits. I also see a dedication among my readers to do so in a safe, natural way while also being mindful of our environment. This book offers me the opportunity to share some ways hydrogen peroxide is used to promote good health and well being.

My mail also shows that you have many unanswered questions about how hydrogen peroxide cleans, how it can be used around the home and what part it plays in maintaining a healthy body. As always, my first consideration in bringing cleaning tips and remedies to you is:

- Could this do harm?

- It is safe?

- Is it time tested?

- What are the benefits?

- What are (if any) potential problems?

Beyond that, much of what this book does is relate the history of how people across the world, and over the years, have found hydrogen peroxide to be useful in their daily lives.

My fascination with all things natural and kind to the body and environment encouraged me to gather this collection of cleaning and health lore. Many of these hints and tips work wonders – in a particular situation. In other circumstances, they may be less effective. A lot depends on the specific cleaning chore or body concern. I invite you to enjoy reading the cleaning tips and healing remedies in this book to see how others have used hydrogen peroxide.

Over the years we have shared many old time remedies and remembrances of times past. This volume, THE MAGIC OF HYDROGEN PEROXIDE, is another journey into fresh, safe cleaning and time tested healing remedies.

Unlike many of the other natural substances I have written about being used in home remedies, hydrogen peroxide does not have thousands of years of history. It was first isolated in 1818, and was not widely used for many years after that.

Once this remarkable substance did become widely available, its importance as a disinfectant, bleaching agent and all around germ killer made it a popular household staple.

Grandmother used it to remove wax build up from our ears and as a mild antiseptic wash for scrapes and cuts. She even rinsed our toothbrushes in it once in a while to cut down on germs and used it to wipe down her kitchen counters. Little did I know then, that thousands of gallons of hydrogen peroxide were being used around the world in factories and in hospitals for the very same purpose.

And, hydrogen peroxide was rapidly finding a place in both the military and in civilian propulsion research. How, I wondered, could the clear, watery, mild substance I poured over a scraped knee power a rocket or produce an impressive explosion?

A little research solved the problem for me. A heavily diluted solution of hydrogen peroxide such as the 3% solution available at my corner drug store is 97% water and practically harmless.

Stronger solutions are another matter entirely.

In fact, as hydrogen peroxide approaches purity it becomes less and less stable. Depending on how it is produced, it can have small amounts of trace minerals in it. Even if these traces are too tiny to be seen by the naked eye, they are still important to what happens next. At high concentrations, hydrogen peroxide will react with tiny trace amounts of metals and – POOOOF! An explosion occurs.

By controlling the kind and amount of additives to a concentrated hydrogen peroxide solution, a controlled burn can be produced. This results in a very efficient fuel – the kind that was used in the first rockets, such as Germany's infamous V rockets of World War II. Even more important, this is pretty much a non-polluting, renewable fuel. This is the kind of renewable energy source that may be an important part of filling tomorrow's energy needs.

While all this was happening, the medical use of hydrogen peroxide was also expanding. At solutions of 30% or so it is used to sanitize and disinfect equipment in hospitals, clinics and doctor's offices.

Because of hydrogen peroxide's many uses in and around the home, it is a natural addition to our series of books on home remedies and natural healing practices.

Although you cannot grow or make your own hydrogen peroxide, as is true of most of the healing substances we have explored together, hydrogen peroxide is an inexpensive, readily available, easy-to-use liquid.

Like all old-time wisdom that is handed down from one generation to the next, many uses are very helpful today. Still, others may not be the best solution in today's world. Be sure to talk to your healthcare practitioner before making regular use of any home remedy, whether it is hydrogen peroxide, baking soda, vinegar or any other food or substance.

Please remember, this book is an attempt to share information. The proper use of hydrogen peroxide to clean and heal will not disturb the environment, set off allergic reactions, pollute the air we breathe or deliver harsh chemicals to skin and air. But, even this remarkable substance has its limitations. Use it wisely and use it in moderation. And, consider this volume as your open sesame to the incredible, wonder of hydrogen peroxide!

I hope you will join me in the pages that follow and discover, as I have, the many wonders and uses of hydrogen peroxide. Then, please feel free to write to me and share your own experiences with this remarkable natural substance. I look forward to reading about the newest discoveries and personal uses you have found for hydrogen peroxide in your own lives and homes.

Wishing you all the best,

Emily

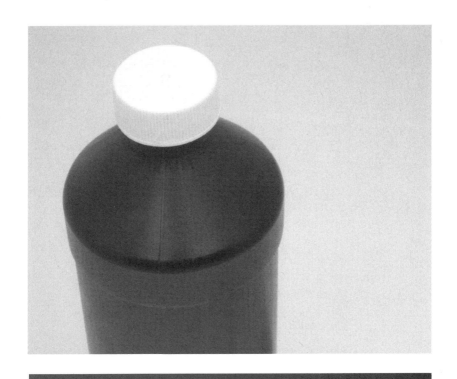

Introduction

INTRODUCTION

Welcome to *The Magic of Hydrogen Peroxide*. *The Magic of Hydrogen Peroxide* is the latest in a series of books by Emily Thacker highlighting common, household pantry staples that can double as both wonderful health remedies and amazing cleaning agents: garlic, vinegar, honey, baking soda, green tea...and now hydrogen peroxide! You may wish to reference the Appendices chapter in the back of this book for a brief description on each of these wonderful books full of home remedies, cleaning solutions, recipes and ways they can positively impact your life and well-being.

So, what could garlic and hydrogen peroxide possibly have in common with each other? One is a chemical molecule; a powerful bleaching agent capable of launching rockets and powering engines. The other, an edible herb closely related to the onion family we use every day to flavor our favorite foods. So, what do they have in common? Both of these share many important, useful factors such as:

- Easily found on your grocer's shelves or in your own kitchen pantry

- Inexpensive

- Natural and safe for the environment

- Can help maintain a healthy, vigorous lifestyle

- Can be a safe, natural alternative to toxic household chemicals

- Can be, in moderation, an important part of maintaining a healthy lifestyle

While hydrogen peroxide shares each of these wonderful attributes, this amazing liquid stands out from its pantry counterparts in a very unique way. While each of my previous books has focused on a substance that has been around for thousands of years, hydrogen peroxide is a relatively new discovery. It has only been thought to have been discovered since the early 1800s, and it would be many more years before hydrogen peroxide's use would become widespread throughout homes and the medical field.

This opens the door to new and amazing uses for hydrogen peroxide to be discovered each and every day! While new uses are constantly being found, many of the remedies and techniques in this book were methods our grandparents and great grandparents relied on generations ago.

Our grandmothers knew so many helpful uses for hydrogen peroxide. She wiped down counter tops and sterilized cutting tools, cleansed cuts and scrapes and disinfected household items. As word traveled of its amazing versatility, everyone from healthcare professionals to beauty consultants began finding new and fantastic uses for this wonderful household product:

- Softening ear wax

- Hair color highlights

- Bacterial killer

- Bleaching agent

- Tooth whitener

- Skin lightener

- Laundry cleaner

- Stain remover

- Wound healer

- Household disinfectant

As hydrogen peroxide's use became more well known, research began into ways of changing the composition and makeup of the agent to suit different uses. As you will discover in reading the history of hydrogen peroxide, this ingenious liquid is available in many concentration grades. Scientists have found that, as the hydrogen peroxide compound itself changes in concentration, so do its many uses.

For example, most of the lower-grade uses of hydrogen peroxide are for consumer use, such as cleaning and disinfecting purposes, or even gardening uses, while the highest grade concentrations are found useful for the military in explosive devices and fuel applications. Plus, there are a multitude of uses for the grades found in between the two.

For clarity sake, unless otherwise noted in this book, we will be referring to 3% hydrogen peroxide grade, the most common form, and that most readily available at your local grocery and drug stores. Remember this grade of hydrogen peroxide can not only be found at your local drug store or grocer in that familiar brown plastic bottle, but also purchased in bulk if you plan on using it widespread. This will not only be more convenient than running to the store purchasing bottles, but also prove to be even more cost effective!

As an example, 3% hydrogen peroxide grade is 3% hydrogen and 97% water, often times combined with some other additive used as a stabilizing agent. Remember that many hydrogen peroxide concentrations use additives to help stabilize this chemical. These agents could be harmful if ingested in large amounts, so remember, do not swallow hydrogen peroxide. If, in your own search for hydrogen peroxide uses, you come across a personal health remedy calling for ingesting hydrogen peroxide, be sure and run it by your own health care practitioner first, just to be on the safe side!

Countless uses for hydrogen peroxide have been documented and handed down through past generations, and all in just a relative few years! But there is still much to be discovered. This book hopes to introduce you to the

amazing uses of yet another wonderful household staple…
and then act as a springboard for hydrogen peroxide
discoveries of your own.

So let this book be a help to you and your family, and
be sure to share discoveries of your own with Emily, too, as
we discover *The Magic of Hydrogen Peroxide* together!

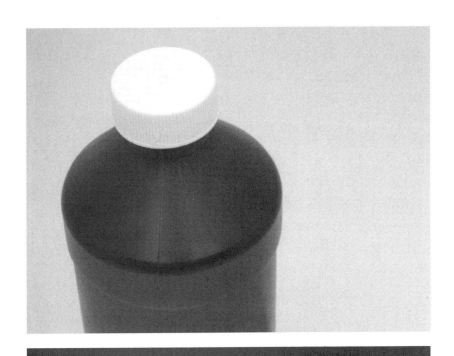

CHAPTER ONE

Hydrogen Peroxide's
Fascinating History

A LITTLE HISTORY

Hydrogen peroxide's history is both very old and relatively new: naturally occurring hydrogen peroxide is formed inside the body by all living creatures and is also created by light in the atmosphere.

Inside the Body

Inside the body, hydrogen peroxide can be very destructive to individual cells. Still, it is impossible to eliminate it, as it is formed when the body breaks down fatty acids and certain amino acids. Every time we eat, some hydrogen peroxide is made by the digestion process. Hydrogen peroxide is also formed in places such as the mitochondria when oxidation occurs.

Some enzymes undergoing oxidation first produce superoxide, then that degenerates into hydrogen peroxide. An example of how superoxide is produced, is when white blood cells encounter harmful micro-organisms. They immediately produce hydrogen peroxide, superoxide and hypochlorous acid. Pretty much, they bleach the invader to death!

The superoxide, a molecule with three oxygen atoms, is very unstable. So, when it comes into contact with liquids, it combines with water and breaks down into hydrogen peroxide.

To limit hydrogen peroxide's destructive properties, each of the body's cells has a small compartment-like area or sac called a peroxisome, where hydrogen peroxide is locked away and stored until it can be broken down by the body's catalase.

Those Pesky Oxygen Molecules

When too many free radical bearing molecules, such as superoxide and hydrogen peroxide, are circulating in the body, they overcome its usual defenses and begin to damage cells. These so-called "reactive oxygen species" (molecules with an abundance of oxygen atoms that are free to readily combine with most everything they come into contact with) are believed to be an important factor in the aging process.

These highly reactive, oxygen-bearing molecules are thought to be responsible for almost all degenerative diseases. This seems to be especially true in the case of Parkinson's disease and, perhaps, some dementias.

Even more distressing is the fact that as free oxygen damage is done to the body, the by-products of this damage are themselves detrimental to the body's cells. The resulting build up of damaged cells accelerates the aging of cells. This vicious cycle continues until the body breaks down entirely.

Alzheimer's disease researchers have found that oxygen related stress markers characterize the neuropathology of the disease. The amyloid related brain damage has been linked to hydrogen peroxide that is naturally produced in the body. Spectro-analysis shows that trapped oxygen molecules react with minute traces of metal, such as iron or copper, to increase the stress on brain cells.

This added stress results in the formation of these plaques that are so characteristic of Alzheimer's disease.

Hydrogen Peroxide and HIV

Medical researchers at Emory University in Georgia have been working with the relationship between HIV and hydrogen peroxide. Preliminary results indicate that when an inflammation occurs in the body, hydrogen peroxide is formed as a by product of the action of white cells. They have shown that this encourages HIV cells to multiply more rapidly than usual. It is thought that the hydrogen peroxide acts as a chemical messenger telling the HIV cells to become more active.

Hydrogen Peroxide and Ovarian Cancer

In a mini version of the hydrogen peroxide and mineral reaction that results in explosions, hydrogen peroxide has been found to be toxic to ovarian cancer cells. Researchers at the University of California at Los Angeles say that hydrogen peroxide is particularly toxic to these tumors when some compounds were present and much less so when others are present. This has led them to the conclusion that hydrogen peroxide both targets and destroys the ovarian cancer tumor cells by way of a metal mediated response. It is hoped that this knowledge will lead to new ways to target cancerous cells and to destroy tumors without doing great harm to surrounding tissue. This is an imperative part of treating the cancer as a whole.

In the Atmosphere

Did you know hydrogen peroxide is found naturally in our atmosphere? Ozone in the atmosphere is made up of three oxygen molecules. Water vapor is made up of two hydrogen molecules and one oxygen molecule. When an ozone molecule is hit by ultraviolet light in the presence of water, one of its three oxygen molecules combines with the water and forms a new compound. This new compound is made up of two hydrogen molecules and two oxygen molecules and is called hydrogen peroxide (H_2O_2).

This new compound is denser than water and has a sharp, mildly acidic odor. It is clear, even in high concentrations. Hydrogen peroxide is often found diluted in water, but is also sometimes diluted in alcohol or ether. Left to itself, it will decompose into harmless water and oxygen.

As the chemical concentrations, or grades, of hydrogen peroxide change, so do its uses. As the concentration grows, so does the solution's strength and potency. At low grade, such as 3%, skin can be affected to a minimal degree. When hydrogen peroxide is in a higher concentrated form, it can blister the skin. As a solution of hydrogen peroxide becomes more and more concentrated, it can even become an important part of an explosive process. Concentrations above about 6% should only be used by those trained in its use and who know proper safety methods for handling it. Some of the most important grades (or concentrations) of hydrogen peroxide and how they are used follow:

3% Most common form, widely available at grocery and drug stores. Used for cleaning simple cuts and scrapes, as well as cleaning and antiseptic purposes.

6% Available at beauty supply stores, used in bleaching and coloring hair.

30% Used in chemical laboratories as a reagent and as a bleach in the manufacturing of textiles and paper.

30% -32% Electronic grade. Also used in the manufacturing of foam rubber.

35% - 50% Technical and food grade. Used in some laboratory experiments and to sanitize manufacturing equipment associated with food processing.

90% - 99% Used in military and fuel applications. It is a high energy, renewable fuel for lightweight engine uses.

BEWARE

Although diluted hydrogen peroxide is a safe, highly useful antiseptic, misuse of it does carry some dangers. Its antiseptic and bleaching qualities cause it to be irritating to delicate mucus membranes. Holding it in the mouth for extended periods of time, or even sniffing it into nasal passages can irritate or burn tender tissue.

The United States Food and Drug Administration warns of serious health risks – even death – associated with the improper use and abuse of hydrogen peroxide.

Great care must be taken in its use.

Hydrogen peroxide does a good job of washing out and disinfecting new scrapes, cuts and abrasions. However, repeatedly applying it can interfere with the healing process itself.

For example, applying hydrogen peroxide to a surgical incision will foam away surface bacteria and help prevent infection. But, it will also affect the healing edges of the incision and discourage them from generating the new growth needed to close the incision properly. For this reason, extended soaking of any wound in this remarkable stuff should, in most cases, be avoided. Always speak with your healthcare provider before using hydrogen peroxide to heal open wounds, particularly after surgical applications.

Hydrogen peroxide has an amazing ability to help reduce minor bleeding in cuts and scrapes, But, according to doctors at Mayo Clinic, too frequent application of hydrogen peroxide to an open wound can allow it to adversely affect blood flow in capillaries. This, in turn, prevents the edges of the wound from knitting together and healing properly.

Direct contact or prolonged exposure to even slightly concentrated hydrogen peroxide can harm the skin. Some of the results of contact with concentrated hydrogen peroxide follow:

- Blistering of skin

- Delayed wound healing

- Skin bleaching

- Whitening of skin

Blood stains on clothes, linens and other textiles can almost always be lifted with hydrogen peroxide, but its bleaching action may also lift any color from the item being treated. Be sure and spot check any areas of fabric to be treated with hydrogen peroxide prior to application.

OXYGEN THERAPY

Intravenous administration of hydrogen peroxide is sometimes advocated as a treatment for a wide variety of health concerns. Three of the most popular ones are for multiple sclerosis, cancer and HIV. The American Cancer Society considers intravenous hydrogen peroxide therapy to be not only unproven but to be actually dangerous.

Injecting hydrogen peroxide has been touted as a way to quickly raise the oxygen levels of the blood. The unfortunate truth is that high levels of hydrogen peroxide in the blood can lead to the formation of oxygen bubbles in the blood stream. Then, these bubbles can actually block and inhibit blood flow. The result is a stroke because normal blood flow is blocked. Or, depending on the location of the block, a limb or digit may become gangrenous. Very serious and dangerous health effects from misuse.

Even if the oxygen released by injecting hydrogen peroxide into the blood stream does not form dangerous bubbles, it is a risky undertaking. Hydrogen peroxide destroys the blood cells responsible for causing it to clot when a person is cut. This makes excessive bleeding a very real danger.

Other advocates of what is usually called 'oxygen therapy' suggest swallowing various amounts of hydrogen peroxide. This, too, is considered by most medical practitioners to be dangerous undertaking and an unacceptable health risk.

Ingestion of hydrogen peroxide, particularly the 35% food grade variety or higher concentrations, can cause harm to the body. Even inhaling the fumes can cause injury to delicate lungs. Internal use of hydrogen peroxide has been linked to:

- Vomiting

- Throat and mouth burns

- Abdominal pain

- Difficulty in breathing

- Seizures

- Stomach damage

- Death

Drinking hydrogen peroxide is especially dangerous for young children. The cancer agency in Canada has issued a special notice warning of the danger to children who may drink this antiseptic.

Hydrogen Peroxide Production
Production of this useful acid can be achieved by several methods. All of these methods have been developed since 1818, when the first hydrogen peroxide was 'discovered' by Louis Jacque Thenard. He burned barium salts to create barium peroxides, which were reacted with nitric acid and dissolved in water. An impure hydrogen peroxide was produced.

Later, the barium peroxides needed for Thenard's process were formed by using hydrochloric or sulfuric acids. But, his general method of producing it was used for more than 50 years, until more modern methods of obtaining hydrogen peroxide were later discovered.

Today, most hydrogen peroxide is produced by what is called the anthraquinones oxidation process. In this process, hydrogen peroxide can be produced by:

- Treating water with ultraviolet light

- Running electricity through water

- Bubbling ozone through cold water

- Treating barium peroxide with sulfuric acid

The purest, highest strength hydrogen peroxide is made through the process of electrolysis.

Hydrogen peroxide has many uses in both chemical laboratories and inside and outside of the body. But inside the body, it has been linked to a wide range of tissue damaging reactions. Naturally occurring hydrogen peroxide has been linked by some researchers to the development of both Parkinson's disease and Alzheimer's disease.

To understand how it can damage the body it is necessary to understand how hydrogen peroxide is formed inside the body. We should also understand how it reacts inside the body.

Hydrogen peroxide is formed by white blood cells in our immune system. It is this production of hydrogen peroxide that grants our immune system the ability to ward off harmful attack.

The hydrogen peroxide chemical compound, H_2O_2, is the water molecule (H_2O) plus the addition of an extra atom of oxygen. Considered an unstable molecule in most circumstances, it is willing to give up its extra oxygen atom fairly easily, freeing an oxygen atom, which is able to roam loose or bond with other elements. These atoms are referred to as free radicals.

The concept of free radicals has been the subject of many news and medical reports in recent years. They have been much talked about in the medical field for some time, considered a probable explanation for many age-related health conditions in everything from Alzheimer's Disease to cancer.

But, free radicals can also be quite beneficial to our body's immune response system against dangerous viruses and bacteria. They do this by oxidizing any foreign invaders to the body.

Oxidation is the free radical oxygen atom attacking bacteria or other invading organisms directly. This attack results in the oxygen ꞌꞌching holes through an organism's protective membrꞌ ꞌctively killing the bacteria.

We know hyd / ꞌoxide, when used as a microbial, is an effective gꞇ acteria fighter. This natural fighter is not only produced within our own bodies, but also in nature itself.

Hydrogen Peroxide in Nature

Honey is one of nature's wonders! Its golden goodness is packed with vitamins, minerals and an amazing array of healing enzymes. It is used in medicine as a wound dressing because of its ability to attract moisture and for its infection fighting powers. One of the reasons it is able to kill germs so well is that it contains hydrogen peroxide, a natural enemy of bacteria.

The special makeup in honey that hold down and inhibit the growth of bacteria are called inhibines. They are, mostly, by-products of glucose oxidase, an enzyme bees add to nectar when making honey.

The glucose oxidase in honey is a fermenting agent. It comes from fungus (much like penicillin does). When honey is eaten, the acid it produces is one of the things that helps the kidneys remove poisons from the body.

Glucose oxidase acts on glucose in unripened honey. It makes gluconic acid and hydrogen peroxide, which are both sensitive to light and heat. This is one reason why the best honey is never exposed to great heat or strong sunlight.

Because hydrogen peroxide is considered to have powerful free radical-like tendencies, it is destructive to healthy cells as well as dangerous cells and is considered by most medical scientists as a strong factor in accelerating aging of the body.

Melatonin and melanin, are involved in regulating the body's coloring pigments and sleep patterns and are strong antioxidants. As such, they are very involved in the chemistry of the body and seem to be a factor in delaying the aging process. It has been found that the hydrogen peroxide formed by cells as they assimilate fats and proteins tends to destroy melatonin. Researchers are working on using this knowledge to delay aging and enhance cell health.

Employing a seemingly contradictory view of hydrogen peroxide, some researchers are advocating its intravenous use as treatment for some medical conditions.

This use of hydrogen peroxide for this purpose is highly controversial, and anyone considering this use should thoroughly research this type of therapy before beginning a course of treatment. This research should include a consultation with your personal medical practitioner or specialist in the field.

HYDROGEN PEROXIDE'S MANY USES

Hydrogen peroxide is widely used as a disinfectant. Its uses range from killing bacteria on simple scrapes and cuts to sterilizing satellites.

One of hydrogen peroxide's very first uses was to bleach the straw used in making hats. Today, more than a billion pounds of pure, 100% hydrogen peroxide is produced every year. It is used in food processing, paper manufacturing, electronics, oil refining, mining and to treat waste water and other industrial wastes.

Manufacturing Uses

Hydrogen peroxide is used to bleach many commercial products. These include:

- Silk

- Straw

- Wool

- Feathers

- Cotton

- Hair

- Wood pulp

- Bones

The Food and Drug Administration has cleared hydrogen peroxide for use in the manufacturing of personal medical devices. It is being found that it is a faster and more efficient method of sterilizing objects than most other methods.

Cosmetic Uses

Cosmetologists and beauticians have long touted the benefits hydrogen peroxide brings to the health and beauty arena. This wonderful solution is an obvious choice to aid in hair highlighting and lightening as well as a tooth whitening agent. It is so popular as a bleaching element it can be found as the whitening ingredient in many over-the-counter tooth whitening toothpastes and kits.

Just a few of hydrogen peroxides cosmetic uses include:

- Hair highlighting

- Hair streaking

- Skin lightening

- Arm hair lightener

- Tooth whitening

- Skin toner and refresher

- Acne fighter

- Age spot remover

- Nail bleaching

- Brow lightener

Food Processing

Hydrogen peroxide is active against both bacteria and mold spores, making it ideal for disinfecting equipment used in food processing. Sometimes it is used at elevated temperatures to increase its effectiveness.

The United States Environmental Protection Agency considers hydrogen peroxide to be an approved substance for sanitizing kitchen utensils, appliances and other food processing equipment. The fact that it rapidly breaks down into plain water and oxygen means that no poisonous chemicals are left behind to contaminate food.

Hydrogen peroxide's lack of toxic residue makes it an ideal rinse for fruits and vegetables. *The Journal of Food and Science* reports that it is even able to kill E. coli on fresh apples!

Treating Waste

Waste management is an ongoing problem that promises to become even greater in the future. Storing hazardous materials merely moves the problem from one location to another. Hydrogen peroxide has the ability to neutralize many dangerous contaminates. It is also encourages many others to break down into harmless compounds.

For example, sulfur containing by-products of many manufacturing processes can be difficult to dispose. Treating them with hydrogen peroxide can help to eliminate their worst traits by changing their chemical composition.

Fuel Cells

Hydrogen peroxide is a clear liquid; at high concentrations it may appear to be slightly light blue in color. In high concentrations it burns skin. In a sense, hydrogen peroxide is pure, concentrated energy. At high concentrations in can explode.

Hydrogen peroxide stores energy in the form of chemical energy. Researchers are working on putting the entire process of producing hydrogen peroxide into small fuel cells that can power cars.

When hydrogen peroxide is used as a fuel, it is not burned in the sense that petroleum based fuel is used and consumed. It decomposes, releasing energy in the form of heat that creates steam and oxygen. This rapid decomposition is channeled into propulsion in a miniature version of the same power used to blast off a rocket. This reaction was used as the fuel for underwater torpedoes during World War II. It is also the reason one should never toss a lighted match into any hydrogen peroxide solution.

Is hydrogen peroxide going to be a reasonable choice in the future for powering cars? Right now, it appears to be a much cheaper and cleaner renewable fuel than petroleum based ones.

Once a production facility is built, hydrogen peroxide can be very cheap to produce. For raw materials, it uses the hydrogen and oxygen that are in the air! This clean, renewable process includes a starter of anthraquinone. This salt is only a enabler. It is recovered at the end of the process and can be used over and over as it is not used up or destroyed. This also helps to keep down the cost of manufacturing hydrogen peroxide.

Hydrogen peroxide engines are expensive to install, especially in today's cars that are pre engineered to run on petroleum based fuels.

In combustion engines, hydrogen and air are used to generate a controlled chemical reaction in a fuel cell. This is how electricity for running the car is generated. Electricity is produced with a by-product of water. The first stage forms H_2O_2 (hydrogen peroxide), the second stage converts the H_2O_2 into H_2O (water).

The entire process converts the hydrogen and oxygen into tremendous power. For example, a test car, powered with hydrogen peroxide, was able to accelerate from 0 to 450 mph in 34 seconds. A true powered jet car!

The Ronn Motor Company, located in Texas, is in the process of producing a car with an onboard fuel cell. Their Scorpion is expected to mix hydrogen fuel with gasoline to result in a very fast, powerful vehicle that should have mileage of about 40 miles per gallon of gasoline. This $150,000 car will have a race car chassis and a six speed transmission.

In the meantime, drag racing already has hydrogen peroxide powered cars up and running. And they are running very fast. These engines mostly work by flooding screens made of platinum or silver with hydrogen peroxide. Instantly, a huge cloud of steam is released out the back of the car and the car is propelled forward at a few hundred miles an hour!

The fuel for these cars is cheap, the speeds are extraordinary, and petroleum based pollution is eliminated. When pure hydrogen peroxide is used as fuel, the only by-products are oxygen and water.

In Madison, Wisconsin, mopeds are also being tested using a kind of onboard fuel cell system.

Others are working on perfecting hydrogen peroxide powered generators, welding machines and self-propelled flying apparatus, including a rocket belt. These new uses include streamlined fuel cells that are much smaller than anything yet in production.

This includes a hydrogen peroxide powered bicycle that reaches incredible speeds. One so called 'rocket bike' is expected to produce nearly a thousand pounds of thrust and there is a 'rocket cart' that will probably develop about three thousand horsepower! There is even a racing car under development that is expected to have a sixteen thousand horsepower engine and reach four hundred miles per hour in a quarter mile!

Hydrogen peroxide fuel may soon power a personal back pack helicopter and fuel cells are under development that will run on sea water and solar energy.

On the Farm

Some farmers believe that hydrogen peroxide has important uses in their fields. This may stem from the fact that this mimics one of nature's best fertilizers, rainwater, which contains a greater amount of hydrogen peroxide than water used in irrigation. It is said that if you spray a dilute hydrogen peroxide solution on:

- **Carrots** – they will absorb more of the nitrogen that is in the air. And, adding sugar to the mix will make the carrots taste sweeter.

- **Alfalfa** – it will grow taller and be more resistant to pests such as weevils and aphids.

- **Green bean plants** after picking off all the beans –, they will bloom again and you will be able to harvest another crop.

- **Garden seeds** – they will sprout in a shorter amount of time and a larger percentage of them will germinate.

- **Tomato plants** – they will thrive and be more resistant to blight and fungus attacks. Sometimes hydrogen peroxide is even mixed half and half with fat free milk and used as a fertilizing spray!

Some controlled studies dispute the belief that hydrogen peroxide soaked seeds sprout faster. But, its ability to kill disease causing viruses and bacteria that may be on the seeds has been proven, so it is very likely that a larger percentage of soaked seeds will survive to germinate. Sterilization with hydrogen peroxide is an especially good way to rid seeds of any spores from powdery mildew and mold. It also helps to prevent dampening off.

Some farmers claim that plants, if treated regularly with hydrogen peroxide, will develop stronger root systems. Some of this belief is based on the fact that hydrogen peroxide is an important part of how plants naturally send signals from one part of the plant to another. Plants increase and decrease the flow of chemicals, such as hydrogen peroxide, to alert the plants' natural protective powers when attacked by insects or disease.

Before using any dilution of hydrogen peroxide on a plant, be sure to test it on a single leaf. Spray it on, wait a few days, then check to make sure there are no harmful effects. Most established plants can tolerate a solution made of half water and half drugstore quality hydrogen peroxide. Never spray hydrogen peroxide on newly emerging crops or on young transplants.

Bleaching

In other hydrogen peroxide news, paper mills that have traditionally used old fashioned chlorine bleach are switching to this less environmental toxic liquid. The mills are finding that when hydrogen peroxide is used to bleach the paper pulp the yield is higher and overall costs are less.

One of the lesser known uses for the bleaching action of hydrogen peroxide is in the field of natural history and forensic medicine. Bones are often bleached with a hydrogen peroxide solution. It does minimal damage to them and is less toxic for researchers.

For personal care, freckles and liver spots will go away if wiped down with a mixture of drugstore hydrogen peroxide and ammonia. As this mixture dries out the skin, disfiguring spots will flake off, never to return. Use with caution on delicate skin!

Medicinal Uses

Because it is a safe topical antiseptic, hydrogen peroxide, as a 3% or stronger solution, is widely used in the medical community. Some of its most well known uses include the treatment and disinfecting of:

- Animal bites

- Broken blisters

- Insect bites and stings

- Sore throats

- Cuts

- Bedsores

- Abrasions and scrapes

One of the safest methods of sterilizing biological safety cabinets and barrier isolators is to use hydrogen peroxide. It has an advantage over some disinfectants because is clear and does not leave visible traces behind. And, its slight odor quickly dissipates. Even more important for many institutions is the fact that hydrogen peroxide is readily available and inexpensive.

Research is always being done in the field of medicine regarding new and effective uses for hydrogen peroxide. There has been a long debate about using hydrogen peroxide intravenously to treat more serious illnesses and medical conditions.

On one side of the debate, hydrogen peroxide is thought to have very serious negative consequences on delicate internal tissue, causing everything from stomach cramping and breathing troubles to seizures and even death.

On the other side, many researchers believe hydrogen peroxide therapies have proved highly beneficial when administered under the watchful eye of knowledgeable healthcare providers.

We have all heard of the body housing both good and bad bacteria. Good bacteria being found in the colon or vagina that works hard to destroy harmful bacteria that has entered the body. One way our body naturally rids itself of harmful bacteria is through white blood cells. These tiny cells naturally produce hydrogen peroxide and use it to magically oxidize any bad bacteria it encounters in our system.

Since we know the oxidation process through which hydrogen peroxide works is deadly on harmful bacteria, many researchers believe there are a host of medical conditions that respond positively with appropriate hydrogen peroxide therapy. A few of these conditions which hydrogen peroxide therapy (mostly intravenous) has been used successfully include:

- Alzheimer's disease

- Allergies

- Cirrhosis of the liver

- Multiple sclerosis

- Influenza (flu)

- Herpes

- Type II diabetes

- Emphysema

- Parkinson's disease

- Lupus

- Bronchitis

- Parasitic infections

- Cardiovascular disorder

- Periodontal disease

- Shingles

- HIV

As promising as these therapies sound, always consult your own healthcare physician before beginning any regimen calling for intravenous or ingestive hydrogen peroxide usage.

Hydrogen Peroxide as a Mouthwash
While strong concentrations of hydrogen peroxide can be damaging to delicate mouth, eyes and throat tissue, dilute mixtures of the solution are often prescribed. Properly used, it is a great way to kill germs and fight infection.

The *Merck Manual* is the 'gold standard' of treatment guidelines for physicians. It recommends using a 3% solution of hydrogen peroxide, diluted half and half with water, as treatment for Trench mouth.

The government's Food and Drug Administration has also given their seal of approval to hydrogen peroxide as a safe substance when properly used. They have approved the use of a 3% solution as a mouthwash.

All of this does not mean that it is recommended to hold hydrogen peroxide in the mouth for extended periods of time. While hydrogen peroxide has been shown effective as a dental rinse and oral antiseptic, Harvard Medical School has warned that extended soaking of teeth in a non diluted solution, may soften tooth surfaces. They also note that overuse might damage skin cells and delicate oral tissue inside the mouth.

Summing Up
The best medical opinions seem to agree that hydrogen peroxide has an important place in the medicine cabinet. But, as with any effective substance, it should be used with restraint and care.

A HISTORY OF HYDROGEN PEROXIDE USE

1863 – Messner proves that hydrogen peroxide is present in rain water. This fact is important in the history of mankind because much of the water early mankind drank was from rain, leading some researchers to wonder if small amounts added to drinking water would be advantageous today. (Other researchers strongly disagree with this conclusion.)

1888 - The *Journal of the American Medical Association* reinforces the fact that hydrogen peroxide had been proven, nearly 25 years previously, to be an ingredient in the rain water earliest man used for drinking, bathing and washing.

1904 – Charles Marchand publishes the last of his series of 18 books on hydrogen peroxide as a treatment for typhoid fever, gastric ulcers, bronchitis and tuberculosis.

1904 – Edmund Nacht proclaims that a 6% solution of hydrogen peroxide is a good disinfectant for the throat. He also suggests its use as a mouth rinse.

1913 – The *Journal of the American Medical Association* reports that hydrogen peroxide is good for killing germs in milk. It goes on to note that the effectiveness of this method of sterilization is dependant on the quality of the milk. For example, the higher the butter fat content, the less effective a set amount of hydrogen peroxide will be.

It is also recognized as a germicide for drinking water. Generally, hydrogen peroxide is considered an emergency treatment for drinking water, as other methods are preferred. (One advantage to hydrogen peroxide may be the fact that with vigorous agitation and exposure to sunlight, it will kill germs and then most of it will decompose.)

1920 – *The Lancet*, England's most respected medical journal, opens the discussion on the value of using hydrogen peroxide as an intravenous infusion.

Breaking with orthodox medical opinion, some doctors suggest that harmful free radicals in the body are not the result of the normal breakdown of food, but are the product of incomplete oxidation during the process. They go on to reason that adding the extra oxygen that makes up hydrogen peroxide will prevent free radicals from building up and causing cells to age rapidly.

1957 – *Nature* magazine reports that replacing the water of cancerous rats with an extremely diluted hydrogen peroxide solution results in about half of their tumors shrinking, some even totally disappearing. When the hydrogen peroxide is discontinued, the tumors do not return. Early tests report possible human cures, too.

1983 – Medical researchers begin work on testing the oral ingestion of hydrogen peroxide to fight disease.

1985 – Tests of hydrogen peroxide as both an oral treatment and as an intravenous infusion to fight disease and tissue degeneration continue. Some work is also beginning on using it as an intra-artery infusion.

The use of both oral and intravenous hydrogen peroxide is very controversial. Standard medical treatment centers do not, in most cases, endorse this practice.

As Fuel and Military Uses

Back in the early 1950's, pilot Scott Crossfield flew into history by piloting the first eight flights of the now-famous experimental X-15 rocket. This amazing, experimental rocket was powered by six small hydrogen peroxide jet engines.

Hydrogen peroxide's ability to release large amounts of energy has made it useful as a fuel. As early as 1971, the British were using it as a rocket propellant. It was also the fuel for the V2 rocket and the Black Knight plane. It has been used to energize:

- Airplanes

- Submarines

- Rockets

- Torpedoes

- Missiles

- Spacecraft

Using hydrogen peroxide to generate energy is a particularly efficient, low cost method. The technology that produces this energy is fairly light weight, making it especially useful in aircraft and spacecraft. It is being developed by the military as a method of generating electrical power.

In the space program, is has been used to sterilize satellites.

For many years, pure, highly concentrated, hydrogen peroxide was thought to be unstable. This is because Thenard's method left traces of solids and heavy metal ions behind. These reacted with concentrated hydrogen peroxide to create what chemists call catalytic decomposition. Most of us know catalytic decompositions by another name. We call them explosions!

Probably the first use of hydrogen peroxide as a fuel was by the German Luftwaffe. During World War II they developed a rocket engine that was powered entirely by a process dependant on hydrogen peroxide. Soon after this, they developed an engine powered by hydrogen peroxide to use in their Messerschmidt planes. Hydrogen peroxide solution was also used to power their destructive V-2 rockets and in submarines and torpedoes. Reusable catapults were also propelled with a hydrogen peroxide solution.

In the years after WWII, the English developed their Black Knight and Black Arrow rockets. They were powered by Rolls Royce engines, using a hydrogen peroxide and kerosene based fuel.

Several kinds of engines that ran on hydrogen peroxide were developed by the American military in the years that followed and were used until jet engine technology replaced them.

An interesting out growth of the hydrogen peroxide rocket fuel experiments was the development of the Personal Rocket Belt by Bell Aircraft Company. Shown at the 1984 Olympic Games in Los Angeles, it immediately became part of futuristic folklore. Since that early patent has now expired, any one who wants to can now make their own!

Rocket grade hydrogen peroxide is an 80% - 98% concentration and must be very free of contaminates. Other names for this grade of hydrogen peroxide include propellant grade hydrogen peroxide and high test peroxide (HTP).

Recreational use of hydrogen peroxide has resulted in some interesting transportation and propulsion devices. Hydrogen peroxide is the fuel of chose for those who need a low weight engine to develop lots of speed during short runs. These include:

- Rocket belts.

- Gyroplanes, such as the 1957 Fairey Rotodyne that could carry about 50 passengers. Researchers in Sweden tested a gyro glider that could make vertical takeoffs in 2003.

- Helicopters, including ones with rotor tip rockets and are back sized.

- Rocket cars.

- Rocket go carts.

- Rocket bikes, such as the one Eric Teboul raced for 50,000 fans in August of 2009.

Nature's Own Hair Bleach

Research from the Federation of American Societies for Experimental Biology has identified hydrogen peroxide as the major agent affecting the graying of hair. According to their research, daily wear and tear on hair follicles allows a build up of hydrogen peroxide in the scalp. This eventually blocks the production of melanin, the natural coloring in hair, leaving hair gray.

Young people manufacture a tiny amount of hydrogen peroxide in hair forming cells. With age, the amount of hydrogen peroxide increases dramatically. Eventually it bleaches the melanin from the hair, from the inside out.

Researchers are now trying to find a way to prevent this natural build up of hydrogen peroxide. An essential amino acid, L-methionine, is one of the preventatives scientists are looking at. It can be found in sesame seeds, soybeans, some nuts, fish, spinach and potatoes. Ongoing scientific investigation is seeking to determine if supplementation with L-methionine has the ability to affect the natural graying process.

Household Mold

The United States Department of Housing and Urban Development includes hydrogen peroxide on their list of approved disinfectants for 'certain biohazards.' This list includes treatment for ridding homes of certain molds that are hazardous to the health of any inhabitants.

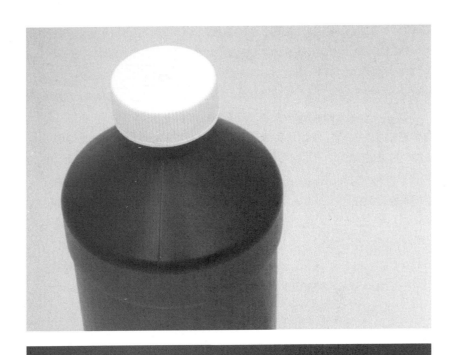

CHAPTER TWO
Getting Started

Look Before You Leap

Before you begin putting to use all the magical uses of hydrogen peroxide, it may be helpful to learn a few important, basic facts. Keep in mind hydrogen peroxide is still a relatively new substance as far as home and personal use is regarded. While many of these remedies and solutions are considered tried-and-true, many should still be tested under the watchful eye of your healthcare professional.

Just use common sense when trying something new or unfamiliar to you. Everyone's body is unique and reacts differently, so listen to what your body is saying to you. A few tips on the generalities and use of hydrogen peroxide will go a long way in making the most of this miraculous solution.

In a Nutshell, What is Hydrogen Peroxide?

Hydrogen peroxide, or H_2O_2, is a viscous liquid, clear or very light blue in color. Viscosity rates its 'flowing ability,' for lack of a better description. Viscous is the ability of a liquid to flow. The higher the viscosity, the slower the liquid's flow. For example, honey is of a higher viscosity than water, therefore it flows slower. Hydrogen peroxide has a slightly higher viscosity than that of water.

Hydrogen peroxide is the chemical formula H_2O_2 (remember back to your school days and studying the atomic chart in chemistry class?). It is basically the water molecule (H_2O) with one additional oxygen atom. Because of this extra atom, hydrogen peroxide can easily and rapidly break down into simple water, losing its extra oxygen atom and safely evaporating back into the air or getting absorbed into surrounding material. And what happens to that missing, extra oxygen atom? It simply dissipates into the air.

Since hydrogen peroxide changes and evaporates so quickly, its water evaporation leaves behind no chemical residue, unlike chlorine bleach, which could be dangerous to people or the environment. This helps ensure hydrogen peroxide will not leave traces of harmful or toxic chemical solutions. Hydrogen peroxide is safe for both humans and the environment.

It is because hydrogen peroxide is so easily changed from H_2O_2 to H_2O that great care should be taken not to leave the peroxide out in the open. If you are, for example, soaking a toothbrush in hydrogen peroxide for disinfecting purposes, keep in mind the peroxide will quickly lose strength and become weaker and weaker.

So remember, for many of these remedies, you will want to use fresh hydrogen peroxide, or consider freshening what you are using each and every time. Setting out in the open air and light quickly causes hydrogen peroxide to lose potency.

Those Great Brown Bottles
It is this very reason hydrogen peroxide is most often sold in those familiar brown bottles. The dark plastic blocks out sunlight which can speed up the disintegration process.

And, hydrogen peroxide becomes less and less potent with age, as it gradually decomposes and morphs into simple water.

So, how do I use this stuff?

Household hydrogen peroxide (3%) can be purchased from most local grocery or drug stores. 6% peroxide can be obtained through many beauty or cosmetology outlets. Higher grades of hydrogen peroxide can be dangerous and difficult to come by, and should probably be avoided.

Hydrogen peroxide degrades very easily, losing potency as it loses its extra oxygen atom. Care should be taken in using and storing hydrogen peroxide to insure longevity.

Prior to purchasing, be sure and check the expiration date on the bottle's label to make sure the solution isn't already past its potency height.

When storing hydrogen peroxide, do so in its original brown bottle (to keep light at bay) in a dry place away from humidity. After opening the bottle, peroxide should last at least six months if stored correctly. If left uncapped or exposed to light, the breakdown will occur much quicker and peroxide will lose potency.

Also be sure not to accidentally introduce contaminants into the bottle itself. This will hasten breakdown. For example, as you are using the peroxide, pour the peroxide into a spoon rather than placing the spoon inside the peroxide bottle. This will keep outside elements from entering the solution.

When using higher grade concentrations of hydrogen peroxide, wear gloves so the solution does not irritate your skin.

As you begin to try hydrogen peroxide remedies, as with any new solution, start small and work your way up. Everyone's body reacts differently and has different outcomes. Make sure you are taking small steps and are satisfied with the results before continuing.

Hydrogen Peroxide and Nature

Because hydrogen peroxide is so close to water in molecular makeup, it is a natural companion to our fragile ecology. The fact that this odorless, colorless liquid contains only one additional oxygen molecule, and that it loses that molecule so easily (turning it into simple water), keeps it safe for riverbeds and streams. Meaning, when you rinse your used hydrogen peroxide down the kitchen sink, you need not worry about it harming the environment. It is also safe for septic systems and leach beds.

Remember

As you are beginning to use hydrogen peroxide, remember to:

- Keep out of the reach of children

- Store in its original container. If you must store hydrogen peroxide in another bottle, be sure to mark it clearly and accurately so everyone can easily read the bottle's contents

- Use protective gloves, if necessary, to avoid potential skin irritations

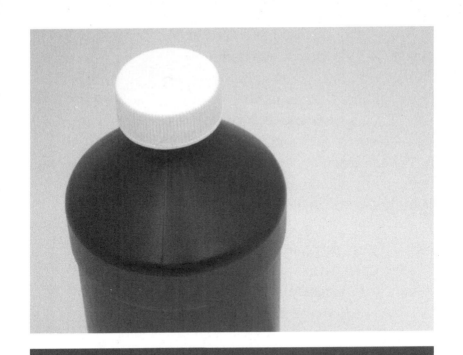

CHAPTER THREE

Hydrogen Peroxide and Better Health

Remember the skinned knees and scraped elbows of childhood? We would rush home to our waiting mothers who quickly patched us up with a splash of hydrogen peroxide and a bandage. Kiss on the knee included! Our mothers knew hydrogen peroxide was both a safe disinfectant for cuts and scrapes as well as a way to help lessen the bleeding. Mom believed in this wondrous healing agent as a safe remedy for simple ailments. So how does hydrogen peroxide actually work on our bodies?

How Does Hydrogen Peroxide Work?

Hydrogen peroxide is a very strong oxidizer, which means it can actually change chemical make up through the fizzing action that occurs while using it. Hydrogen peroxide forms its famous bubbling action when it comes in contact with a catalyst. In the case of cuts and abrasions, or any open wound, that catalyst is an enzyme called catalase. Catalase is an enzyme found naturally in blood (among other places). Those infamous bubbles you see on contact with peroxide are oxygen gases being released.

Hydrogen peroxide works on open wounds by closing off blood vessels and other small capillaries to reduce bleeding through its oxidation process. And, because it is so reactive as an antioxidant with the amazing ability to actually change the components of many known substances, hydrogen peroxide works fabulously as a disinfecting agent.

When hydrogen peroxide comes into direct contact with bacteria, its oxidizing action begins, rendering some of the bacteria's components useless. This produces holes and tears in the bacteria's delicate membrane. That membrane acts as a defense barrier, and when it becomes damaged the bacteria is killed off and dies. This makes hydrogen peroxide not only a miraculous disinfecting agent, but also a powerful antimicrobial solution as well.

HYDROGEN PEROXIDE IN THE HEALTHCARE FIELD

For more than 100 years, hydrogen peroxide has been used by hospitals and clinics as a disinfecting agent. Because of its unique ability to zone in on blood residue and quickly neutralize any germ agents that are present, hydrogen peroxide solutions have been depended on to keep patient areas and treatment instruments safe and sanitized. You can find the solution being used in:

- Hospitals

- Clinics

- Emergency rooms

- Stat care rooms

- Assisted living centers

- Veterinarian offices

- Dentist offices

- Physician and doctor offices

- Nursing homes

- Preschools

- Child care centers

All have trusted the effectiveness of hydrogen peroxide for years. They have depended on this amazing solution for sterilization and disinfecting of:

- Patient tables

- Operating rooms

- Counter tops

- Triage areas

- Delicate surgical instruments

- Patient areas

- Dental tools

- Hazardous spills

Even though hydrogen peroxide's history has been relatively short, it has proven itself indispensable in the medical field. So, it is no surprise to find that for generations we have used this miraculous product at home as a safe, gentle home remedy for many of our own personal health care needs.

Just remember, please don't ingest or swallow hydrogen peroxide without first consulting a physician, as some grades can be harmful. Your own personal physician will be able to help guide you through some of your questions as to how hydrogen peroxide can be beneficial to your particular circumstance.

Here are just a few helpful suggestions to get started discovering how versatile hydrogen peroxide really is. I am sure you will discover even more as you make hydrogen peroxide a part of your own health routine.

Migraine Headaches

Studies have shown that migraine headaches can be relieved in as little as just a few minutes with intravenous hydrogen peroxide therapy. Researchers believe the addition of hydrogen peroxide into the blood stream causes blood vessels to dilate in cerebral arteries, lessen the affects of migraines. The same remedy is currently being tested on transient stroke patients and so far, the results are promising.

Mouthwash

Take a mouthful of hydrogen peroxide and rinse it around your teeth and gums to help keep your mouth fresh, clean and free of germs.

As you experience the foaming action that occurs with using hydrogen peroxide as a mouthwash or dental rinse, remember it is ridding your mouth of bacteria with each fizz!

Gargle with a mouthful of hydrogen peroxide diluted in water and then rinse for a cleaner, fresher mouth.

Toothpaste

Combine hydrogen peroxide and household baking soda together to form a thick paste. Brush teeth and rinse well.

Homemade hydrogen peroxide toothpaste will not store well for long periods of time before it begins to lose some of its effectiveness. So, be sure and mix together small batches at a time.

Soak your toothbrush in a dish of hydrogen peroxide to kill germs and keep bacteria from forming on bristles.

Toothaches

Have a bad toothache? Pour two capfuls of hydrogen peroxide in your mouth and swish around affected tooth for 5 – 10 minutes. Pain will lessen and bacteria around tooth will be eliminated.

Dental cleaning solutions

Adding diluted hydrogen peroxide to your dental pick and spraying your gums will further rid your mouth of unwanted bacteria between the teeth and around the gum line.

You can also brush your teeth with hydrogen peroxide diluted 50% with water.

Mix ½ teaspoon baking soda with ½ teaspoon hydrogen

peroxide for a powerful tartar remover in between visits to the dental hygienist.

In between teeth

To help remove tea or coffee stains from teeth, try brushing in a 50/50 hydrogen peroxide and baking soda solution for one week. Some people have even added a pinch of salt to this solution for greater stain removal.

Fight gum disease

Make a gum disease fighting paste by mixing hydrogen peroxide and baking soda into a creamy paste. Using your fingers, massage paste into gums, both front and back. Rinse clean without swallowing paste. This will help keep your gums healthy and free of disease.

Fight periodontal disease by rinsing gums weekly with hydrogen peroxide.

Gingivitis can be avoided by swishing a few capfuls of hydrogen peroxide and water around the mouth.

Dental appliances

Soak dental appliances, such as retainers or night brace mouth pieces, in a solution of hydrogen peroxide and water to keep them germ and bacteria free.

Occasionally disinfect small brushes used to keep braces clean in a bowl of hydrogen peroxide.

Dentures

Keep dentures clean and fresh by soaking in a solution of hydrogen peroxide and water a couple of times per week.

Gargle

Safely eliminate germs and bacteria by gargling daily with a few tablespoons of hydrogen peroxide. This will rid your mouth of germs while leaving teeth and gums fresh and clean.

Mouth ailments

Hold a tablespoon or so of hydrogen peroxide in your mouth for a few minutes each day to prevent mouth and canker sores from developing.

Treat irritating mouth ailments, such as canker sores or denture sores, with a treatment of hydrogen peroxide. Rinse your mouth several times a day with a 50/50 solution of hydrogen peroxide and water to help lessen or cure the ailment.

For irritations left from orthodontic appliances like braces or retainers, gently rinse mouth daily with hydrogen peroxide solution diluted with tap water.

Botulism

Botulism is a serious illness brought about by the Clostridium bacteria. This bacteria can enter the body through contaminated food or infected wounds. A 3% hydrogen peroxide is sometimes used to treat wound botulism.

Dogs suspected of eating contaminated carrion are sometimes treated by immediately inducing vomiting with hydrogen peroxide. Be sure and consult a veterinarian right away if you suspect your pet has eaten something that could carry the botulism bacteria for instructions on how to safely induce vomiting.

Digestive Problems

Some say that digestive problems, particularly those brought on by food borne illness and bacteria, can be eased by ingesting a low concentration of diluted hydrogen peroxide. Normally very small, diluted amounts are taken over the course of a few days, with relief coming within a few days. But, great care should always be taken if you are considering ingesting hydrogen peroxide. Always speak with your physician first, as severe throat and stomach burns or vomiting can occur when ingesting hydrogen peroxide in high concentrations.

Antibacterial hand cleaner

Wash hands in hydrogen peroxide to rid hands of bacteria after working outside, in the garden or around animals.

Hydrogen peroxide makes a wonderful hand disinfectant to keep germs from spreading to newborn babies.

Soak hands in hydrogen peroxide diluted with water after touching blood or fecal matter to rid them of possible germs.

To rid hands of both germs and strong odors, wash

them with a mixture of hydrogen peroxide and baking soda until the smell dissolves away.

Cuts and abrasions
Splash a little hydrogen peroxide on simple cuts, scratches and abrasions to kill germs and fight infection.

Hydrogen peroxide can be sprayed onto skinned knees for tender relief in little ones.

Do not use hydrogen peroxide on deep tissue cuts or wounds, as this will hamper the delicate healing process.

Rashes
Use hydrogen peroxide as an antiseptic for rashes by gently dabbing rash area with a cotton ball or soft cloth soaked in hydrogen peroxide.

Using a spray bottle, spray hydrogen peroxide onto rash to disinfect.

Deodorant
Spray hydrogen peroxide under arms for an inexpensive deodorant. Peroxide eliminates bacteria growth that causes underarm odor.

Hydrogen peroxide can be blotted under arms with a moistened cloth or cotton balls to use as a deodorant.

Ear cleaner
To clean your ears, simply add hydrogen peroxide to

your ear and allow to fizz. Tilt your head to allow used peroxide to leave the canal and repeat with other ear.

Wipe outside and backs of ears with a soft cotton ball soaked in hydrogen peroxide for a finishing clean.

Ear aches and infections

Using a dropper, tilt head and gently administer hydrogen peroxide to affected ear. Keep hydrogen peroxide in ear for a few seconds until bubbling and fizzing action subsides. Tip head to empty used hydrogen peroxide onto a paper towel or tissue.

For a nasty ear infection, pour hydrogen peroxide into ear canal and allow to rest for about 45 seconds. Empty ear of peroxide. Repeat twice a day, if necessary.

Put a drop or two of hydrogen peroxide in your child's ear at the first sign of infection to keep earaches at bay. Be sure and prepare your child in advance for the fizzing sound he is going to hear!

Ear itching

End itchy ears by pouring hydrogen peroxide into itching ear. Keep head tilted, holding peroxide in ear, for about 30 – 40 seconds. Tilt head in the other direction and empty out peroxide. This should end the itching.

Ear wax

Gently and safely remove built up ear wax with hydrogen peroxide. First, carefully pour some hydrogen peroxide into ear canal and tip your head to keep solution from exiting.

Leave peroxide in your ear until bubbling action stops, usually 20-30 seconds. With a clean syringe or straw, gently pour warm (not hot) water into ear canal to flush out wax. For heavy wax, repeat 2 – 3 times a day until clean.

Remember that some wax in your ear is good. You are only trying to remove the excess build up.

Loosen ear excess ear wax by filling the ear canal with hydrogen peroxide and allow bubbles to fizz and subside. This lets you know it is working to clear away wax. Then, simply drain peroxide from ear canal and blot the outside of the ear clean.

Foot odor
Soak feet in a bath of warm water and a few cups of hydrogen peroxide to relieve feet of foot odor. Soak for a few minutes several times a week.

Athlete's foot and other problems
Soak feet in a warm solution of hydrogen peroxide and water for 5 minutes per day. Dry feet with a soft towel.

Spray the inside of shoes with undiluted hydrogen peroxide and allow to air dry to keep athlete's foot from festering.

Spray a coat of undiluted hydrogen peroxide on the floor of your shower to help eliminate athlete's foot fungus.

Upon checking into your hotel room, spray shower stall area with hydrogen peroxide to eliminate any fungus-causing germs that may be lingering. Pay close attention to the bottom area of the stall.

After showering in a public shower such as a hotel or pool, spray or wipe down the bottoms of your feet with hydrogen peroxide to prevent a fungal infection from beginning.

People say that soaking your feet in a warm bath of half hydrogen peroxide and half water will kill foot fungus. Be sure and let feet dry naturally.

Boils and blisters

Do your feet have painful boils or blisters? Prevent infection while promoting healing by soaking feet in a warm pan of water and hydrogen peroxide. Solution works well if you combine a cup or two of peroxide with a gallon of water. Soak for 20 – 30 minutes every night. Rinse feet and pat dry with a clean cloth.

Arthritis

Soaking in a warm tub with a cup of food grade hydrogen peroxide is also good to ease the complaints of arthritis sufferers.

A quarter cup of hydrogen peroxide can also be added to a warm foot bath to help ease arthritic joint pain.

Rheumatism

Many long time sufferers of rheumatism believe that soaking in warm hydrogen peroxide baths help ease symptoms of the disease. Try adding between one half cup and one full cup of food grade peroxide to warm bath water. If food grade peroxide is not readily available, you can substitute drugstore 3% grade, but it would take two or three bottles to reach the desired consistency. Once peroxide is added to the water, take a restful soak for 20-30 minutes to ease discomfort.

Fibromyalgia

Fibromyalgia is health condition affecting millions of Americans. Studies have shown that stimulating the body's immune system can be very beneficial in treating fibromyalgia. There are many natural methods for jump starting the immune system such as eating a well-balanced diet rich in fresh fruits and vegetables, avoiding stress and adding supplemental vitamins to your diet.

Another way of stimulating the body's immune system for fibromyalgia sufferers is by increasing the amount of oxygen found in the body. There are many easy and natural ways to begin increasing oxygen in your body, such as keeping a free flow of fresh air into your home; increasing gentle exercise; practicing deep breathing routines; stimulating body massages. Several methods of increasing oxygen levels in the blood involve the use of hydrogen peroxide. Again, suggested remedies differ widely, but are worth mentioning. Some users have begun by simply adding a cup or so of hydrogen peroxide to warm bath water and soaking the body a few times per week. Other remedies include the addition of hydrogen peroxide to a vaporizer or beginning a regimen of intravenous hydrogen peroxide therapy under a physician's supervision. Be sure and consult a knowledgeable physician about the benefits of hydrogen peroxide therapy. If you are unsure about qualified physicians in your area, a list of physicians and agencies specializing in hydrogen peroxide therapy can be found in the back of this book.

Clogged Arteries

Research is beginning to show that intravenous hydrogen peroxide therapy can also be used in the treatment of clogged arteries and cardiovascular disease. It is believed that the introduction of hydrogen peroxide and its unique oxidative properties into clogged arteries may actually help dissolve arterial blockage. While many of these studies are still quite new, results so far have been promising. Research is also being done into the effects of hydrogen peroxide into vascular muscle.

Nail problems

Kill fungus on your fingernail bed by soaking nails in hydrogen peroxide for a few minutes a day. Be sure to rinse clean and dry. Repeat as necessary.

Eliminate toenail fungus by soaking feet in a hydrogen peroxide and water bath twice a day. Fill a pan half full of warm water and half full of hydrogen peroxide. Soak for 5 – 10 minutes. Rinse and dry feet. Repeat for one week, or until toenail fungus is gone.

Rid yourself of unsightly yellow nail fungus by soaking fingernail or toenails in a pan of water and hydrogen peroxide.

Foot bath

For a wonderful treat for your feet, soak in a warm foot bath once a week. Simply pour a cup of hydrogen peroxide into a warm foot bath. You can also add a few drops of perfume or oil as appreciated.

Soaking in a hydrogen peroxide foot bath once a week can help kill any bacteria on your feet and prevent the start of athlete's foot or other fungal infections.

Resting your feet for just a few minutes a day in a warm, hydrogen peroxide bath can help prevent, reduce or eliminate toenail fungus.

Clean between toes to rid feet of athletes foot by blotting with a cotton ball or soft cloth doused in hydrogen peroxide. Allow toes and feet to air dry completely before putting on shoes or socks.

Be sure and clean all your foot gear with hydrogen peroxide to keep germ free:

- Toe nail clippers

- Pumice stone

- Nail brush

- Foot cloths

- Toe separators

Body soak

For a refreshing body soak, add 2-3 cups of hydrogen peroxide to your warm bath water. Remember, hydrogen peroxide will cool your bath water's temperature, so be sure and pay close attention to water temperature as you fill your tub!

Add a handful of Epsom salts or a splash of your favorite body oil to your hydrogen peroxide bath for a beautiful soak.

Place a cup or so of hydrogen peroxide in your bath water for skin conditions such as boils, fungus or other infections.

Body wash

Hydrogen peroxide is a wonderful bacteria-fighting antiseptic that kills bacteria lingering on the body's skin. Remember to wipe down daily, or as needed, for fresh, germ free living.

Keep a bottle of hydrogen peroxide in a spray bottle. Spray body while in the shower and rinse clean.

Body aches

Some people say soaking in a warm bath with a cup or two of hydrogen peroxide added will ease sore muscles and chronic joint pain.

Bedsores

Painful bedsores can be relieved by dabbing a soft cloth or cotton ball dampened with hydrogen peroxide over the sores. The fizzing action of the bubbles will begin to work on lessening the sores.

Compresses made by soaking a clean cotton cloth in hydrogen peroxide diluted in cool water and placed on the irritating sores can also help ease bedsore pain. Leave compress in place for 10 - 15 minutes before removing. A clean compress should be used each time.

Animal bites
Bites from animals run the risk of infection. Pour hydrogen peroxide solution over a bite from an animal to disinfect area immediately from bacteria or germs. This will also help reduce bleeding. Wrap area with a clean, soft cloth.

Pet scratches
Use a light s\   of hydrogen peroxide to wipe down a pet scrat   stant relief.

Insect bites
Keep a small   le of hydrogen peroxide in your purse or car for a quick remedy for insect bites.

Blot bites from mosquitoes or stings from bees with a cotton ball or tissue dampened in hydrogen peroxide.

Disinfect the bite and prevent infection from mosquito bites with a quick spray of hydrogen peroxide. Keep a small spray bottle in your purse or car to have with on hikes or picnics.

Enema

Mix 1 tablespoon of hydrogen peroxide to two cups of distilled water to make a homemade enema solution.

Yeast infections

Rid the body of yeast infections by douching with a solution of hydrogen peroxide and water mixed to a 1:3 ratio. For example 1 tablespoon hydrogen peroxide (3% grade) to 3 tablespoons warm water.

This method of treatment for yeast infections can be highly argumentative, as some people feel douching is never necessary. Some physicians believe that because the body makes its own hydrogen peroxide along with other good bacteria, douching should be avoided. You may wish to consult your health care professional on the benefits of douching.

Colds

Fill your nostrils with a solution of half water, half hydrogen peroxide. Hold for a few seconds and blow out to rid yourself of sinus infections and cold symptoms at the first sign of illness.

Sore Throats and Colds

Find yourself coming down with a cold or suffering from a sore throat? Try gargling with a mouthful of drugstore grade hydrogen peroxide to end sore throat pain. You can also place a teaspoon or so of hydrogen peroxide into your ear canal, wait a few moments, and let drain out to keep away ear infections that may accompany your sore throat or cold. For added relief, try adding a little peroxide to your nasal inhaler, too.

Ease breathing difficulties

Add about 2 cups of hydrogen peroxide to each gallon of water in your humidifier. It is a method to gently deliver hydrogen peroxide to your respiratory system during breathing flare ups.

Asthma

Asthma sufferers may find relief through hydrogen peroxide therapy. The thought behind treatment is to improve the body's immune system and while adding the benefit of extra oxygen to the body. The addition of hydrogen peroxide to the body in aerosol form can be one way to accomplish this. Adding hydrogen peroxide to a humidifier can be one way to introduce the remedy easily into the respiratory system. This can not only raise the level of oxygen in blood stream, but also increases efficiency of the immune system.

One note about adding hydrogen peroxide to a vaporizer or humidifier. Because heavier levels of hydrogen peroxide can be used as a bleaching agent, be sure and keep the vaporizer or humidifier away from delicate curtains or walls.

Allergies

Adding a small amount of hydrogen peroxide to your humidifier or vaporizer can help ease allergy symptoms. Nasal pumps, which can be purchased at a local drug store or pharmacy, can also help distribute a hydrogen peroxide and water solution to help with ease of breathing during difficult periods of asthma or allergy inflammation.

A LITTLE DEEPER HYDROGEN PEROXIDE THERAPY

A Relatively New Science with Promising Results

The subject of intravenous (IV) and oral treatment therapies are one of the most controversial aspects of hydrogen peroxide, but also one of the most intriguing and promising. Hydrogen peroxide's benefits to the medical community have been long documented with great success. It is the question of whether hydrogen peroxide should ever be taken internally that remains a subject of great debate among leading scientific researchers and physicians. Opinions on this subject range from being completely benign and useless or even potentially harmful, to being the single greatest medical discovery in our lifetime.

So what is all this talk about hydrogen peroxide therapy? First, a little background.

The Idea Behind the Science

Hydrogen peroxide not only occurs in nature, but is produced in our own bodies. It is a critical element that our bodies manufacture through white blood cells. It is this production of hydrogen peroxide that grants our immune system the ability to ward off harmful attack.

The hydrogen peroxide chemical compound, H_2O_2, is the water molecule H_2O plus the addition of an extra atom of oxygen. This molecule is considered somewhat unstable, in that it is willing to give up its extra oxygen atom fairly easily, freeing an oxygen atom.

When single atoms are roaming loose and free in the body, they are referred to as 'free radicals.' The concept of free radicals may sound familiar to you. They have been much talked about in the medical field for some time as the probable reason for many age-related health conditions such as:

- Degenerative diseases

- Cancer

- Arthritis

- Diabetes

- Alzheimer's disease

- Ocular diseases

- Parkinson's disease

But, free radicals which are produced in our bodies through white blood cells are also responsible for protecting our body by attacking viruses and bacteria. They do this by oxidizing the intruder, and are a vital part of how our body works to defend itself.

Remember when we discussed how oxidation works? Oxidation is the oxygen atom attacking bacteria or other organisms directly. This attack results in the oxygen punching through an organism's membrane effectively killing the bacteria.

Do you recall as a child how your mother pumped lots of vitamin C into your body at the first sign of illness? Vitamin C actually produces hydrogen peroxide in the body. It is a naturally prevalent element in our colons and vaginal tracts as the good bacteria which wards off infection.

We know hydrogen peroxide as a microbial is an effective germ and bacteria fighter. And, peroxide is more than willing to give off its extra oxygen atom through oxidation.

So, the question remains, how is all of this information beneficial to our health? Is it possible to harness the power of hydrogen peroxide and administer what, if any, benefit it possesses for certain conditions and illnesses?

How Hydrogen Peroxide Therapy Can be Useful

Research into the idea of using hydrogen peroxide in treating patients with chronic disease has been extremely promising. For example, patients suffering from emphysema have responded extremely well to hydrogen peroxide therapy. Sufferers have been successfully treated using both intravenous (IV) therapy as well as inhalation methods. With the inhalation method, hydrogen peroxide is administered through the use of a vaporizer or humidifier. Both with positive results.

Research is showing that hydrogen peroxide therapy can be helpful in treating patients with a multitude of illnesses and maladies. Promising results have been shown in a wide variety of illnesses including:

Allergies
Altitude Sickness
Alzheimer's Disease
Anemia
Angina
Arthritis
Asthma
Bacterial Infections
Bronchitis
Cancers
Candidiasis
Cardiovascular Disease
Cerebrovascular Disease
Chronic Fatigue Syndrome
Chronic Obstructive Lung
    Disease (COPD)
Chronic Pain Syndrome
Cirrhosis of the Liver
Diabetes
Digestion Problems
Emphysema
Epstein-Barr Virus
Erythematosis
Fibromyalgia
Fungal Infections
Gangrene

Gingivitis
Headaches
Heart Arrhythmias
Hepatitis
Herpes Simplex
Herpes Zoster (Shingles)
HIV Infections
Influenza
Insect Bites
Lupus
Migraines
Mononucleosis
Multiple Sclerosis
Pain of Metastatic Cancer
Parasitic Infections
Parkinson's Disease
Periodontal Disease
Peripheral Vascular
    Disease
Prostatitis
Reynard's Syndrome
Rheumatoid Arthritis
Shingles
Sinusitis
Viral Infections

So, why is hydrogen peroxide so promising?

Why Does it Work?

Researchers believe patients not only receive oxygen through the free radical hydrogen peroxide releases as oxygen, but also through a more indirect approach. For example, the oxidation process itself may dilate constricted blood vessels in emphysema patients, causing an increase in oxygen production on its own. For patients who are experiencing chronic breathing difficulties, this could be an incredible, possibly live-saving breakthrough! Any improvement concerning the oxygenation of red blood cells improves a crucial part of lung function. Something vital to those who suffer from the disease.

"For patients who are experiencing chronic breathing difficulties, such as asthma patients, this could be an incredible, possibly live-saving breakthrough!"

Increased levels of oxygen in the bloodstream have been shown effective in:

- Dilating blood vessels resulting in increased oxygen in the heart and brain

- Increasing glucose levels in diabetic patients

- Maintaining good working function of the thyroid

With all these benefits, one can see why breakthrough research of hydrogen peroxide therapy is so crucial. It can give patients otherwise resigned to suffering through their condition hope for a better, healthier life.

Because of the many benefits hydrogen peroxide therapy brings to the body's circulatory system, such as dilating blood vessels and increasing oxygen levels, researchers believe this relatively new method might be a promising way to treat a variety of diseases and maladies. Studies are finding that the addition of the free radical hydrogen peroxide releases in the body can be a beneficial addition to treatment regimens for patients suffering from diabetes, rheumatism, arthritis, fibromyalgia, some forms of cancer, and many breathing ailments such as asthma or emphysema. Studies are also showing that hydrogen peroxide therapy not only improves the immune system, but also helps combat or prevent allergies. There are also added benefits of reducing inflammation.

Bio-oxidative therapies, such as hydrogen peroxide therapy, introduces a new level of oxygen into the body which is believed to increase brain function in patients suffering from various forms of dementia, such as Alzheimer's disease. This increase in oxygen levels may increase cognitive function in helping patients think clearer.

Patients who are suffering from a host of these chronic illnesses, and are not responding well to traditional medical treatments, may want to look into the alternative therapy of hydrogen peroxide bio-oxidative treatments.

Oral Treatment Versus IV Therapy
The decision to begin hydrogen peroxide therapy, whether oral, IV or even inhalation, is one that should be discussed with your health care provider, and if necessary,

a specialist in the field. A physician knowledgeable in the field of peroxide therapy is in the best position to evaluate a patient's condition and determine which course of treatment might be most beneficial.

Everyone's body reacts differently to treatment methods. Hydrogen peroxide therapy is no different. Some conditions respond better with oral therapy while others respond better to IV therapy. Patients can discuss with their doctor why one treatment may work better than another.

More to Consider
While the potential benefits of hydrogen peroxide therapy sound promising, some researchers are not as convinced. Some even go as far to say the therapy could be potentially harmful to the body, and the potential for misuse is present. Hydrogen peroxide therapy is not for everyone, but many patients believe the option is well worth at least looking into.

Patients who have chosen to pursue hydrogen peroxide therapy have noted several potential side affects anyone considering treatment should be made aware of. A specialist familiar with the treatment can advise potential patients on the full range of side effects and potential dangers. A few of these include:

- Sleeplessness when therapy is administered in the hours before bedtime (researchers believe this is due to extra oxygen in the blood stream)

- Nausea and upset stomach (oral therapy)

- Unpleasant aftertaste (oral therapy)

These are just a few side effects to consider when beginning alternative therapy treatments. But many patients believe the positive aspects of hydrogen peroxide therapy greatly outweigh any possible short term, negative side effects. This is something you can discuss with your doctor prior to pursuing treatment.

However, there are a few things that can be done to lessen these side effects. Some of these are relatively simple ideas.

For example, when taking oral therapy, be sure not to eat immediately prior to your treatment time. Hydrogen peroxide combines with whatever food you have undigested in your stomach. Any bacteria or other catalase base (such as potato, etc.) will react with the peroxide solution resulting in its normal foaming reaction. This foaming reaction could prove very uncomfortable and result in upset stomach, nausea or vomiting. Just holding off on administering oral treatment until a recent meal has had a head start leaving the stomach may reduce chances of stomach upset.

Hydrogen peroxide therapy techniques can be a promising option for people suffering many chronic illnesses. Be sure and consult your doctor, or a specialist in the field of peroxide therapy, to determine if this course of action might be right for you.

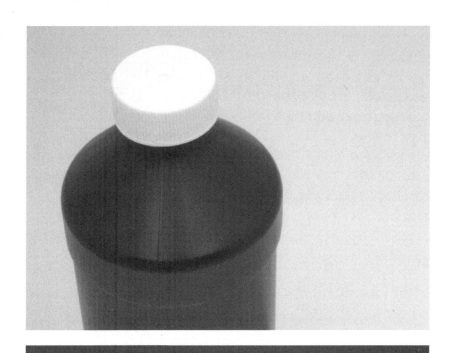

CHAPTER FOUR

Beauty, Skin Deep

Hydrogen peroxide is found naturally in the environment, as well as in our bodies, making it a perfect health and beauty agent for our skin and body. It is delicate on the skin, if used sparingly, and can be diluted with ordinary tap water for a host of uses.

Used for many years by beauticians and cosmetologists, hydrogen peroxide can be found as the chemical lightening agent in many expensive commercial skin and hair lighteners, as well as facial creams. This wonderful solution has proven itself effective as a beauty agent in a myriad of personal applications.

We are all familiar with the idea of lightening hair or adding sun streaks with hydrogen peroxide. But, it is well documented uses go far beyond just coloring hair.

Hydrogen peroxide is a powerful oxidizer and bleaching agent. Through its oxidizing process, hydrogen peroxide works to bleach and lighten whatever it comes into contact with. From fabrics and paper to skin and hair, hydrogen peroxide can, over time, bring amazing lightness and revival to dull or washed out features. This makes it indispensable to beauticians and cosmetologists.

With the cosmetic industry making millions of dollars each year from skin lightening, hair coloring and even cosmetic dentistry practices, we can use this very knowledge at home in our beauty regimens. Why pay hundreds of dollars per year for beauty services you may be able to replicate at home for pennies on the dollar, or even less!

Hydrogen peroxide is both inexpensive and easy to access. A few of the amazing cosmetic uses it has been linked to include:

- Hair lightening

- Age spot removal

- Brow or arm hair lightening

- Skin lightening

- Skin toning

- Nail whitener

- Teeth whitening and restorer

A Few Things to Remember

As you begin to experiment with a few of these new regimens you are about to read, be careful not to drip or spill hydrogen peroxide onto clothing, particularly with peroxide of higher grades. The same lightening action you desire on your hair or teeth could unknowingly wind up on a favorite shirt or blouse. Likewise, be careful not to splash hydrogen peroxide into your eyes. If this happens, quickly flush eyes with cool water for at least 15 minutes to prevent potential damage to delicate eye tissue.

Because hydrogen peroxide is a bleaching agent, and bleaching agents can be drying to the skin (particularly with repeated or prolonged usage), consider using a skin lotion or moisturizer to keep skin soft and supple after your hydrogen peroxide treatment.

Too much hydrogen peroxide also has the ability to dry out delicate hair follicles. You may wish to add moisture back into hair with a follow-up conditioning treatment to leave hair bright and luxurious.

Coming into contact with higher grades of hydrogen peroxide (like the 6% grade used for cosmetic hair bleaching) can cause the skin to turn white on contact. One can avoid this irritation by wearing protective gloves while using the solution. If you find that your skin does become irritated after coming into contact with fresh hydrogen peroxide, immediately rinse the peroxide off your skin by flushing with cool water for a few minutes. After rinsing, skin may still turn a chalky white, but will return to its natural pigment shortly after rinsing.

Be extra cautious when using hydrogen peroxide to treat acne. Peroxide can be a wonderful solution to keep germs and bacteria from building up on the face. This bacteria can be one of the causes for an acne outbreak, or make existing acne flare ups worse. But while using in moderation is fine, prolonged treatment can have the opposite effect and cause permanent skin scarring.

Most of all, have fun discovering new and exciting ways hydrogen peroxide can be added to your beauty routine. Don't obsess about getting rid of every age spot or having the brightest, whitest smile on the block. Each of our features is what makes us unique individuals! Just have fun with it!

Now let's get started!

Tooth whitener

Swish a mouthful of hydrogen peroxide around your teeth and gums once or twice a day. You should see whitening in about a week.

Brush your teeth with hydrogen peroxide to strengthen and whiten teeth, as well as keeping gums healthy.

Use hydrogen peroxide as an after-brushing mouth rinse each time you brush to whiten teeth.

Tooth whitening toothpaste

Make your own whitening toothpaste at home by using hydrogen peroxide and a little fresh baking soda found right in your own cupboard. Mix small amounts of hydrogen peroxide and baking soda until it forms a soft paste. Brush twice a day with whitening paste, being careful not to swallow any of the solution. Rinse.

Make your own ultra tooth whitening tray and paste. Using aluminum foil, form a "tray" that fits around your upper teeth, fitting over both front and back of teeth. Mix your own whitening solution consisting of baking soda and hydrogen peroxide until a very soft consistency, like pudding. Using a toothbrush, apply cream to teeth. Add a small amount to foil "tray" and apply tray to teeth. Keep in place 5 minutes. Brush teeth and rinse clean. Repeat over next 2 or 3 days for whiter teeth.

To remove stains between teeth from coffee, teas or

colas, soak a piece of dental floss in 3% hydrogen peroxide and floss between teeth. Follow flossing with a rinse of hydrogen peroxide to finish the treatment.

Arm hair

Lighten hair on arms or legs by spraying with hydrogen peroxide and blowing dry with a hair dryer. Repeat over several days for lighter hair.

Use a cotton ball dampened in hydrogen peroxide and wipe over arm or leg hair. Allow to air dry, and repeat every day for one week.

You can also spray hair with hydrogen peroxide before sun bathing, allowing the sun to help dry and lighten hair.

Lighten hair

Use a little hydrogen peroxide on wet or dry blonde hair to slowly lighten or add highlights.

Simply spray hydrogen peroxide on hair, and brush through with a comb or brush. Allow peroxide to dry on hair. Wash hair with regular shampoo. You may wish to use a conditioner to help keep moisture in the hair follicles.

Fill a clean spray bottle with hydrogen peroxide and spray throughout hair. For all-over lightening, remember to spray underneath hair as well. Comb through and leave on hair for 1 hour. Wash with shampoo and rinse clean. Follow with a moisturizing conditioner.

Hair streaking (sun streaking)
Want that beautiful, natural look of sun streaked hair any time of year? Hydrogen peroxide is a wonderful means of adding beautiful sunlight streaks to your hair.

Brush hair nicely so you are able to easily see areas you wish to streak. Holding desired section of hair in one hand, take a cotton ball wet with hydrogen peroxide in opposite hand and wet through hair. It is okay to let go of hair once it is saturated and allow to touch other hair areas. Allow to dry for one hour and shampoo peroxide out of hair. You can do several areas of hair at the same time. If you wish to lighten the same area even lighter, reapply peroxide to the same area over the next couple of days, until you reach the desired effect.

Here's another idea for a more naturally highlighted, summer look. Take an eyebrow brush and dip into beauty grade (6%) hydrogen peroxide getting it very saturated. Brush peroxide onto hair in desired streaking areas with eyebrow brush, continually rewetting the brush. Let set on hair for 60 minutes. Wash with shampoo and rinse thoroughly. (6% hydrogen peroxide, in beauty shop terms, is referred to as 20 volume peroxide.) You may wish to wear protective gloves with any remedy using higher grade peroxide to prevent hands and fingers from whitening.

Eyebrows
Lighten dark eyebrows easily with household hydrogen peroxide. Wet eyebrows lightly with water. Using a cotton ball moistened with hydrogen peroxide, gently rub into eyebrows. Allow to air dry or sit in the outside sun for a few

minutes. Repeat as necessary until brows reach desired lightness.

You can also use an eyebrow brush to apply hydrogen peroxide directly to brows you wish to lighten. Be careful not to apply to skin area around brows, as skin may also lighten.

Lip hair
Hide dark hair above the lip line by dousing with hydrogen peroxide and allowing to dry. Repeat as necessary.

Skin
Bring back the natural beauty of young, light skin with this natural face mask. Mix 1 tablespoon of sour cream with 1 teaspoon hydrogen peroxide. Work into facial skin by gently rubbing in circular motions. All to rest on face for 10 minutes and rinse away.

Age spots
Remove age spots by applying hydrogen peroxide to spots before going to bed at night. After several nights, the spots will be lightened or gone altogether!

Soak a cotton ball in hydrogen peroxide and dab onto age spots. Allow to air dry.

Apply a blot or two of hydrogen peroxide and lemon juice onto age spots each night before bed and they will slowly fade away.

Freckles

Lighten freckles by a daily dab of hydrogen peroxide. Allow face to air dry and repeat as desired.

Skin imperfections and toning

Hydrogen peroxide can be used to gently and safely lighten skin imperfections. Blot skin once a day in areas needing a more even tone. Continue until area has reached desired effect. As with many antiseptic toners and cleansers, hydrogen peroxide can be drying to the skin. The use of a moisturizing cream is recommended to keep skin soft and prevent drying.

Remove orange or brown blotches from self tanners

Blotches left on the skin from self tanning solutions can be easily and quickly evened out and removed. Dip a cotton ball in hydrogen peroxide and wipe on the over-colored area. Leave on for 15 – 20 seconds and wipe clean with a second cotton ball or tissue.

Acne

Prevent acne by swabbing your face once a week with hydrogen peroxide. The peroxide will remove any bacteria build up on the face and neck that may contribute to acne growth.

For a breakout of acne, clean your face once a day with hydrogen peroxide and water to remove bacteria on skin that inflames acne.

Need to remove a pimple or whitehead? Gently pop pimple. Wipe clean with small amount of hydrogen peroxide. You will see bubbling action begin as peroxide starts to clean the wounded area. This method should only be used infrequently, as it can irritate or scar the skin if overused.

Wipe face down with light coating of hydrogen peroxide to help dry up pimples.

Dab a little hydrogen peroxide on clear skin to help oxidize the pores and keep skin free of pimples and blackheads.

Dark underarm skin
Lighten dark skin beneath your arms by patting daily with hydrogen peroxide.

Nails
Gently soak fingernails in a bowl of ½ cup warm water, ½ cup hydrogen peroxide and a few drops of your favorite moisturizing hand soap to lighten and brighten fingernails. Rinse and dry when finished. Repeat treatment, if necessary.

Eliminate the yellow tinge left on fingernails after red nail polish use. Soak fingernails in hydrogen peroxide for a few minutes. Wipe clean with cotton ball or tissue, rinse and wipe dry.

Rid toenails of that yellow look by soaking in a foot bath once a day. Mix a 50/50 solution of water and hydrogen peroxide and soak for 5 minutes. Repeat daily until toenails return to a lighter, natural look.

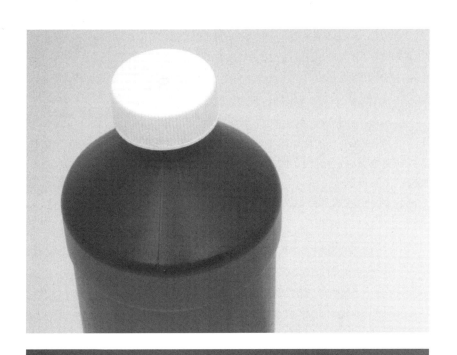

CHAPTER FIVE
Around the Home

So much attention has been placed on hydrogen peroxide's medicinal and cosmetic uses it would be easy to overlook its cleaning and disinfecting benefits. That would be an unfortunate slight.

Hydrogen peroxide's natural antiseptic qualities make it a perfect match for cleaning and disinfecting the household. And, it is readily available in your local grocery or drug store for just pennies on the dollar.

Hydrogen peroxide's ability to quickly kill bacteria makes it an obvious choice for ridding your home of harmful bacteria. Once hydrogen peroxide comes into contact with bacteria, its oxidation process begins.

Oxidation consists of hydrogen peroxide attacking the bacteria and rendering it defenseless through a series of holes in the bacteria's membrane. These rips and holes in the membrane cause the bacteria to killed off very quickly. That is why hydrogen peroxide is considered an antimicrobial agent.

Hydrogen peroxide is considered an unstable chemical molecule, meaning it has the ability to rapidly change compositional make up. This unique trait works to our advantage.

After the hydrogen peroxide has done its job oxidizing and killing off toxic or harmful bacteria, its own decomposition begins. Through contact with air and light, as well as other contaminants, the peroxide itself starts to break down and turn into simple water and oxygen. And, unlike most store bought cleaners, evaporates cleverly and cleanly away, leaving no harmful or toxic residue behind. As we all know, both oxygen and water are found in abundance in nature and are beneficial to the environment in which we live.

This makes hydrogen peroxide a magical cleaning alternative to commercial cleaners and disinfectants. While there are a multitude of cleaners on the market today to clean and disinfect every surface imaginable, most of these can leave behind a chemical residue. That residue can build over time, and even cause sickness after prolonged use. Not to mention the potential damage harmful chemicals can do to our environment as they wash down sinks and drains into riverbeds and landfills. Hydrogen peroxide is a welcome addition to streams and waterways and it degrades into totally natural oxygen and water.

Consider how many different commercial products we purchase to clean and disinfect our homes at any given time. Hydrogen peroxide can replace:

- Bleach

- Tub and shower cleaner

- Mildew spray

- Laundry pretreater

- Tile and grout cleaner

- Oven cleaner

- Antibacterial treater

- Antimicrobial sprays

- Toilet bowl cleaner

- Window cleaner

- Disinfectant sprays

As each of these work to clean and disinfect, these products may actually leave behind their own harmful chemical residue throughout our homes:

- On counter tops

- In baths and shower stalls

- Even on cups and dishes

Hydrogen peroxide can tackle each of these jobs but leaves behind no adverse chemical residue. It all evaporates away as harmless water and oxygen. You can't get much more natural than that!

Hydrogen peroxide's anti-bacterial quality makes it an obvious choice as an effective, inexpensive household cleaner for your kitchen and living areas. But, it gets even better! Hydrogen peroxide is also naturally tough on mildew, fungus and mold making it the perfect choice for cleaning all of your home…not just the kitchen. Tub and shower stalls can benefit from the magical disinfecting power of hydrogen peroxide as it rids your bathroom of grime and germs. Basements can be rid of harmful mold.

Hydrogen peroxide's versatility makes it an obvious cleaner of choice because of traits such as:

• Hydrogen peroxide is found naturally occurring in the human body and in nature itself. It is safe for plants and animals.

• Non-toxic

• Anti-fungal

• Anti-bacterial

• Anti-mildew

• Natural bleaching agent

• Inexpensive

• Leaves no residue

• Readily available

• Replaces countless commercial cleaners

- Environmentally friendly – most cleaners eventually wind up going down the drain or toilet and into sewage systems, and eventually back into the water supply. Since hydrogen peroxide is non-toxic and environmentally safe, it will not harm the water supply, fish and fowl or fragile ecology.

- Safe for people, pets and plants

As you begin replacing commercial cleaners with the power of hydrogen peroxide, your list of amazing cleaning uses around the home will grow and grow!

And, hydrogen peroxide is very cost-effective as a household cleaner, costing just a small fraction on the dollar of what regular store bought cleaners cost. Larger jugs of hydrogen peroxide can also be purchased at even greater savings.

Hydrogen peroxide's oxidation quality makes it a natural bleaching agent with most substances it comes into contact with. It can rid unsightly stains on everything from tile grout to your favorite blouse.

Because peroxide carries bleaching tendencies, care should be taken when using this product. Remember wear protective gloves if contact with the peroxide will be prolonged or if using a grade higher than household (3%). If your skin should come into contact with hydrogen peroxide and your skin becomes irritated, dry or turns a dusty white color, flush skin with cool water for several minutes.

Care should also be taken not to splash hydrogen peroxide onto areas in which you do not wish whitening or bleaching to take place...like that new pair of jeans you just purchased. And always remember to test new fabrics or carpet for color fastness before spot treating or laundering stains with hydrogen peroxide. Better safe than sorry!

Be sure to never splash hydrogen peroxide into delicate eye tissues, or rub eyes with hands that have come into contact with the solution. If contact is made, immediately flush eyes for 15 minutes with cool water.

Planning Ahead
Simple cleaning solutions can be made ahead of time and stored for future use. You will find a few of these referred to in the pages ahead! Feel free to make these solutions and have them on hand the next time you reach for a cleaner at home!

For instance, you can make your own disinfectant spray for both the bathroom and the kitchen ahead of time, always keeping it on hand for when a need arises. Take a clean, plastic spray bottle and fill with hydrogen peroxide. Be sure and label it as such, and place in a cupboard, away from light, to be stored until needed to clean kitchen counters, spray bacteria from garden vegetables or disinfect a cutting board.

Make a second spray bottle to keep on hand in the bathroom. Spray the shower floor when exiting to rid the floor of fungus, or spray down a mirror to keep clean.

Here are a few more cleaners and sprays you can make ahead of time.

Glass cleaner

To make your own glass cleaner, try mixing 2 ½ cups hydrogen peroxide into 1 gallon of tap water. Add 2 or 3 drops of your favorite dish soap and mix. You can pour this into an empty, discarded glass cleaner bottle or pick up an inexpensive spray bottle at the dollar store.

Anti-bacterial spray

Empty a bottle of 3% hydrogen peroxide into an unused spray bottle. Use spray straight and undiluted as an anti-bacterial spray for counter tops and door knobs. Just spray a thin spray of solution on area to be cleaned and wipe with a paper towel, sponge or clean cloth.

This cleaner can also be used to rid your home of bacteria, fungus, mildew and mold!

Hydrogen peroxide's uses are endless! Let the cleaning begin!

KITCHENS

Counter tops and door knobs

Fill a spray bottle with half and half hydrogen peroxide and water to keep on hand to disinfect kitchen.

To deep clean counter tops and door knobs following an illness outbreak in your home, spray with hydrogen peroxide anti-bacterial spray and allow to set for about 5 minutes before wiping clean with a soft cloth. Don't forget kitchen drawer knobs, too!

Prepare two bottles of cleaner: one with hydrogen peroxide and the other with white vinegar. Spray vinegar over area to disinfect. Follow with a spray and wipe of hydrogen peroxide for thorough cleaning and disinfecting of kitchen counter tops and cutting boards.

Soak a kitchen dish cloth in hydrogen peroxide to sanitize counter tops and appliances.

Kitchen sinks and drains
Clean stainless steel sinks and fixtures by spraying with hydrogen peroxide diluted in water and buffing to a high shine with a soft cloth.

Remove any rust on kitchen sinks by spraying with hydrogen peroxide, then sprinkling over with baking soda. Rub into rust stain and allow to set for 10 minutes. Wash clean with a soft cloth.

For difficult stainless steel stains or food that is stuck on, clean with a solution of hydrogen peroxide and a little water mixed with baking soda. Gently scrub stains in a circular motion until clean. Rinse and buff to a beautiful shine.

Periodically rinse a little hydrogen peroxide down the kitchen drain to keep it fresh and bacteria free.

If you have a garbage disposal, you may wish to rinse hydrogen peroxide down the drain along with a little baking soda for extra freshness.

Don't forget to wash your used hydrogen peroxide down the drain. It gives the peroxide one last use before getting rid of it.

Cutting boards

Wipe down and disinfect cutting boards and butcher's blocks with a solution of hydrogen peroxide mixed with white vinegar.

Kill salmonella and other food-borne bacteria by washing cutting boards and butcher's blocks with hydrogen peroxide.

Decontaminate wooden or plastic cutting boards in between switching from meats to vegetables by thoroughly cleaning with a spray of hydrogen peroxide and a good scrubbing.

Always keep a spray bottle of hydrogen peroxide on hand to disinfect cutting boards between chopping meat and other ingredients. You can wipe down kitchen utensils as well.

Trash cans and waste bins

Spray a little hydrogen peroxide on the inside and outside of kitchen trash cans and waste bins to eliminate bacteria.

Dishes

Add a few tablespoons of hydrogen peroxide to your dishwasher's regular detergent cycle for brighter, cleaning dishes. Great for getting drinking glasses sparkling clean, too!

Clean plastic bottles and food storage units by washing with hydrogen peroxide and water. Rinse well with clean water and dry.

Find an old sports water bottle with a mildew smell? Try filling it half full of hydrogen peroxide and half water. Put the cap on and shake. Leave overnight. In the morning, wash clean.

Appliances

Ovens can be made clean again with hydrogen peroxide. Make a thick paste of hydrogen peroxide, vinegar and baking soda. Use to scour the inside of ovens to remove baked-on foods and stains. Don't forget to clean the oven doors, as well.

Adding hydrogen peroxide to your dishwasher will also help keep the unit fresh and clean smelling without mildew or odor buildup.

Keep bacteria from foods by periodically washing inside refrigerator and shelving with hydrogen peroxide and water.

You can pour used hydrogen peroxide down the kitchen drain for one last use killing germs in sinks and basins.

Fruits and vegetables

Rid delicate fruits of insecticides and pesticides by spraying with hydrogen peroxide, and rinsing thoroughly with water. Strawberries are notorious for harboring dangerous chemical residue and should be cleaned prior to eating.

Eliminate wax from the outside of grocery store fruits and vegetables. Soak fruit or vegetables in a sink of cold water and about a half cup of hydrogen peroxide. Rinse and dry.

Soak vegetables in a clean sink filled with cool water and a cup of hydrogen peroxide to kill any bacteria before eating or cooking.

Did you know hydrogen peroxide is an effective solution to combat the E. coli virus on fruits and vegetables? If E. coli is suspected on produce, wash thoroughly in a bath of hydrogen peroxide to kill any of the bacteria. Rinse clean and enjoy!

Keep a spray bottle of hydrogen peroxide handy in the kitchen to spray on vegetables from your garden to rid of any bacteria. Rinse well before eating.

Vegetables and fruit can be washed clean prior to eating or cooking by spraying with hydrogen peroxide diluted in water. Fruits and vegetables can also be soaked in a bath of cool water with a splash of peroxide. Rinse clean and food is now ready to be eaten, free of germs and bacteria.

Remove pesticides in fruits and vegetables by spraying with hydrogen peroxide and rinsing in cool water.

Add about a half cup of hydrogen peroxide to a clean kitchen sink filled with cool tap water. Gently soak fruits and vegetables for a few minutes to remove any dangerous pesticide residue prior to eating. Lightly rinse clean before eating.

Kitchen utensils and cutting instruments
Wash dirty kitchen utensils in a bath of hot soapy water with about a cup of hydrogen peroxide. This will wash away germs and bacteria that may linger on serving spoons and cutting instruments.

Kitchen appliances
Wipe down and disinfect kitchen appliances after each use to keep kitchen area germ free.

Occasionally run a cup or so of hydrogen peroxide through your coffee maker and dishwasher to keep them clean and disinfected. It's an eco-friendly way to sanitize! Note: Be sure to rinse your coffee maker well after sanitizing.

Wipe down the inside and outside of the refrigerator with hydrogen peroxide to disinfect from germs or meat residue such as salmonella.

Clean a microwave oven, both inside and outside, with a few squirts of hydrogen peroxide.

Dishes

Add a few tablespoons of hydrogen peroxide to your electric dishwasher detergent for greater cleaning and disinfecting strength.

Sports water bottle cleaning

Open your plastic sports water bottle and notice that moldy smell? Pour in ¼ cup hydrogen peroxide and swirl around. Rinse with clean water.

For tougher odors or to combat the presence of mildew, pour ¼ cup hydrogen peroxide in water bottle and swirl around. Leave overnight and wash out all the mold and mildew smell!

LIVING AREAS

Mirrors and windows

Spray hydrogen peroxide slightly diluted in water on mirrors and windows and wipe to a clean shine.

Use straight hydrogen peroxide for streak free windows and mirrors.

Wipe down windows with glass cleaner made from hydrogen peroxide.

Also remember to wipe down window sills and edging where moisture can build up causing mold to grow.

Cleaning windows with hydrogen peroxide will make for streak free, shiny windows.

Floor cleaner
Dirty floors can not only be cleaned to a shine, but also disinfected with hydrogen peroxide. Fill a cleaning bucket with 1 gallon hot tap water and add about 2 cups of hydrogen peroxide.

You can also mix warm water and hydrogen peroxide at a 1:1 ratio for an everyday floor cleaning solution. Begin with ½ gallon of water and ½ gallon hydrogen peroxide.

To remove very soiled or greasy spots on kitchen floors, spray hydrogen peroxide solution directly on affected area and wipe clean. This will not only remove the hard to clean spot, but also disinfect from any lingering germ residue. For tougher grease stains, treat a second time and allow peroxide to rest on stain for 5 minutes before wiping clean.

Carpet cleaning solution
Make your own carpet cleaning solution instead of purchasing an expensive commercial cleaner. Simply mix about 2 cups hydrogen peroxide solution with 1 tablespoon liquid soap and enough hot water to fill your carpet cleaner or steamer's reservoir.

For very dirty carpets, try using boiling water in the place of hot water. Be careful when removing and dumping your cleaner or steamer's dirty water reservoir, as the dirty water solution will still be extremely hot.

Carpet stain remover

Use hydrogen peroxide to remove stains on carpet. You may wish to test a small, out of the way area of carpet for color fastness before treating large areas.

Simply spray hydrogen peroxide onto the stained area of carpet and allow to remain undisturbed for 5 or 10 minutes. Take a damp sponge or cloth and soak up the peroxide as well as the unsightly stain. Be careful not to rub the stain deeper into carpet fibers by pressing down. Instead, use a soft cloth or paper towel to pat stain up and soak the stain into the cloth or towel. Repeat if necessary.

For tough stains, spray or pour hydrogen peroxide onto stain. Sprinkle a light coating of baking soda on stained area and allow to set for several minutes. Wipe or vacuum soda powder away.

Clean and disinfect areas of your rug or carpet where vomit has ended up. Spray generous amount of hydrogen peroxide on affected area and sprinkle a light coating of baking soda. Allow to stand undisturbed for 5 or 10 minutes. Remove any large pieces and sweep up or vacuum any visible pieces that remain. Blot clean with damp sponge soaked in peroxide diluted in water. Repeat if necessary.

Clean carpet areas where pets have had accidents to remove any ammonia smell still left behind. The ammonia smell may cause pets to return to the same area time after time.

BATHROOMS

For a general bathroom cleaning, keep a spray bottle filled with 1 cup hydrogen peroxide and 1 cup tap water. Clean as needed to keep bathroom areas tidy and germ free.

Showers and tubs

Keep a handy spray bottle full of half and half water and hydrogen peroxide solution in the bathroom to disinfect on a daily basis.

Spray undiluted (3%) hydrogen peroxide onto shower stalls and tubs. Allow to set undisturbed for 20 minutes and wipe clean.

Immediately following a shower, spray stall down with hydrogen peroxide and water solution, with close attention being paid to the shower floor, to keep fungus or other bacteria from forming.

Be sure and clean soap dishes and shower caddies with hydrogen peroxide to keep clean and scum free.

Clean old bathtubs new again with regular washings in hydrogen peroxide.

For greater, deeper cleaning and whitening of bathtubs, clean with hydrogen peroxide and allow to stand for one hour prior to rinsing clean. Repeat if necessary.

Spray hydrogen peroxide directly onto shower heads and let rest for 10 minutes before rinsing clean. This will keep fungus and mildew from building up on the shower head.

Shower curtains
Wash old shower curtains in the washing machine along with your regular detergent plus a cup of hydrogen peroxide.

Soap scum
Wipe soap ledges clean with straight hydrogen peroxide to prevent soap scum buildup at least once a week.

Hot tubs and saunas
Hot tubs and saunas can be safely and effectively disinfected by wiping down regularly with hydrogen peroxide solution.

Toilets
Pour 1 cup hydrogen peroxide into the toilet bowl and allow to set for 15 minutes. Brush clean and rinse away.

Spray hydrogen peroxide on rim and lid of toilet bowl and wipe clean with a sponge or paper towel to clean and disinfect.

Spray and wipe handles to disinfect and clean.

Tile and Grout
Clean unsightly tile grout by mixing hydrogen peroxide, baking soda and salt into a thick paste. Brush paste into

stained grout and allow to stand for 10 minutes. Rinse with clean water and allow to dry.

Remove stains from ceramic tile. Gently clean tile with a cloth dipped in hydrogen peroxide. You can add a touch of baking soda to the cloth for stubborn stains. Rub stains in a circular motion until removed and clean again.

To rid bathroom tiles of mold or mildew, spray undiluted hydrogen peroxide solution onto grimy area and allow to set for at least 45 minutes before wiping clean. Repeat process, if necessary.

Mildew
Mildew in your bathroom? Remove by spraying with hydrogen peroxide. Allow to stand for a few minutes and then scrub and rinse clean.

For heavy mildewed areas, after spraying with peroxide, try scrubbing sprayed area with a sponge or cloth soaked in baking soda.

LAUNDRY

Peroxide in place of bleach
Hydrogen peroxide can be used in place of bleach when laundering white clothes. Simply pour peroxide into your washing machine's bleach reservoir and launder your white clothes as usual. Clothing will come out white and bright, without the harsh chemical additive of using bleach.

Add about a half a cup of hydrogen peroxide to your laundry's rinse water for whiter, brighter white clothes.

Add a half cup of hydrogen peroxide to your laundry's wash water for cleaner, brighter clothes. Do not add directly onto fabric, unless you want a spot particularly brightened.

Pretreater

Pretreat laundry whites with a few sprays of hydrogen peroxide before washing.

Pretreat and remove underarm stains in white garments by spraying thoroughly with hydrogen peroxide and allowing to stand 10 minutes prior to washing.

Ink stains

Get rid of ink stains in clothing by pretreating with hydrogen peroxide. Spray onto stain and rub very gently into fabric. Allow to stand 5 or 10 minutes before laundering.

Dishrags and towels

Disinfect kitchen dishrags and towels by washing in hot water with a cup or two of hydrogen peroxide added to your regular washing machine detergent. Dishcloths and rags will come out smelling new again, void of that mildew smell that can accumulate.

Wash old, smelly kitchen sponges new again by soaking in a bowl of hydrogen peroxide and water overnight. Rinse and squeeze out to dry to bring new life to an old sponge.

Mildew smell in clothing

To rid your clothes of mildew smell, add 2 cups of hydrogen peroxide to laundry water with detergent and wash as normal.

For mold on clothing, spray the moldy area with hydrogen peroxide and then wash with regular laundry load. You may wish to test a small area of fabric before spraying a large area to test for color fastness.

For cloth items with widespread mold, soak cloth in undiluted hydrogen peroxide for 15 -20 minutes before washing in washing machine. Again, be sure and test fabric to make sure hydrogen peroxide doesn't lighten the fabric, as it is a bleaching solution. Diluting the hydrogen peroxide with water will help lessen fabric fade or color change.

Diapers

Add a few cups of hydrogen peroxide to your washing machine when washing baby's dirty cloth diapers. This will not only help clean and disinfect, but also rid diapers of any lingering smell leaving only a fresh remnant behind.

Baby's Toys

With a spray bottle full of a 50-50 water-hydrogen peroxide solution, squirt down plastic baby toys and wipe clean to keep germs at bay. You can also use this same solution to wipe down baby's high chair and eating tray, as well as plastic bibs and pacifiers.

Red wine stains

Dab generous amount of hydrogen peroxide on stained

area with a sponge or cotton ball. Gently rub peroxide into fabric stain and allow to rest for several hours.

Blood Stains

Hydrogen peroxide is the cleaner of choice for removing blood stains in clothing. Pour a saturating amount of peroxide over blood stained area. Area will begin to bubble blood stain away. Let soak for several minutes before washing as usual.

Tough blood stains can be removed by soaking stain in 1:1 hydrogen peroxide and water. Soak for about 20 minutes and wash as usual.

AROUND THE HOME

Rejuvenate mops and cleaning supplies

Make old cleaning supplies, like mops and rags, new again by soaking overnight in a bucket of hydrogen peroxide mixed with water.

Using hydrogen peroxide as a general cleaning solution around the home will automatically keep mops, sponges, rags and anything else it comes in contact with free of bacteria, germs and odor.

Houseplants

Spray a solution of 1 cup hydrogen peroxide and 1 cup tap water onto houseplants every day. This will help them grow lush and lovely.

Once a week, spray houseplants with a 50/50 solution of hydrogen peroxide and ordinary tap water to keep dust from accumulating.

Have you ever gone away on vacation only to come back to wilted and limp houseplants? Freshen them with a peroxide bath. Spray hydrogen peroxide onto leaves and soil to oxidize them back to health.

BASEMENTS AND GARAGES

Moldy walls
Rid your basement and garage of harmful toxic mold by dousing with hydrogen peroxide.

Spray the moldy area with hydrogen peroxide BEFORE attempting to scrub clean. (Mold is very dangerous to your health. Care should be taken not to breathe in mold spores. **Spraying the moldy area before scrubbing will help keep mold particles from flying around and then being inhaled.**) Allow hydrogen peroxide to remain on the moldy area undisturbed for 5-10 minutes and wipe walls clean with a damp sponge.

For deeper mold stains, wet moldy area with hydrogen peroxide and allow to settle for a few minutes. Prepare a bucket of hot water mixed with a few cups of hydrogen peroxide. Using a sponge, clean area by washing wall in a circular motion. Rinse clean.

PET CARE

Clean animal "accidents" by spraying area clean with hydrogen peroxide and blotting clean. By using hydrogen peroxide instead of an ammonia-based cleaner, animals are less likely to return to the smell and make the same "mistake" again. This trick works with both cat and dog urine.

Wash pet's plastic or stone water and dinner bowls in hydrogen peroxide.

Clean and disinfect animal cages with hydrogen peroxide and allow to air dry.

Small cuts and abrasions on your pet can be cleaned and disinfected with hydrogen peroxide, just like humans. Pour a small capful onto a pet cut and allow to air dry. For more sensitive areas, like the ears or head, drench a cotton ball in peroxide and dab onto the area. Be sure not to use on deep cuts, and be careful not to get the peroxide solution into your pet's delicate eyes.

Clean animal transport crates with a quick douse of hydrogen peroxide.

During water changes, fish tanks can be cleaned out from algae buildup and slime by washing with hydrogen peroxide. Be sure and rinse well before refilling tank.

Clean pet's ears at the first sign (or smell) of infection with a capful or two of hydrogen peroxide. Be prepared, your pet may not be accustomed to the fizzing sound in their ear!

Does your dog or cat have wax buildup in their ear? Here is a simple solution. Pour a little hydrogen peroxide in the ear while holding your pet. Try not to let him shake the peroxide out of his ear for at least 30 seconds, longer if he can handle it. Rinse the ear with warm (never hot) water. Be sure and wipe the inside of the ear with a soft cloth or cotton ball to remove any wax that falls out there. Repeat, if necessary.

Wash pets in a warm hydrogen peroxide bath to rid them of pet odor as well as giving them a good, disinfecting cleaning. Combine about ¼ cup of hydrogen peroxide for every gallon of water you wash your pet in.

Rid Pets of Parasites and Bacteria

Fill a spray bottle halfway with regular tap water. Then fill the rest of the bottle with regular, drug store grade hydrogen peroxide, creating a 50-50 peroxide-water solution. Spray down your infected pet and rub thru his fur and into his skin, being careful to completely avoid the eyes. Wash and rinse your pet thoroughly, just as you normally would. You can even add a few splashes of hydrogen peroxide to your pet's bathwater, again being mindful to keep solution away from delicate eye tissue. Be sure and rinse thoroughly.

Birds

Spray down bird cages with hydrogen peroxide and wipe clean to disinfect.

For metal cages, be sure and wipe completely dry to prevent rusting.

Clean out water trays for bird cages by soaking in hydrogen peroxide for 10 minutes. This will kill any bacteria on the dish. Wash clean and rinse and dry well. This is not for use on metal watering dishes, as this can hasten rust formation.

Cats

Rid the kitty litter box of that lingering smell by cleaning with hydrogen peroxide. Empty litter from box and spray bottom with hydrogen peroxide. Rinse out with garden hose and wipe clean.

Be sure and clean your cat litter scoop by soaking in hydrogen peroxide as well.

Disinfect a cat's abscessed fighting wound with a quick douse of hydrogen peroxide. Be certain the peroxide makes it all the way down to the skin, instead of laying on top of the cat's coat of fur. You may wish to repeat treatment the following day, depending on the severity of the wound.

If you are scratched by your cat, or if your cat has been scratched by another, a few squirts of hydrogen peroxide should clean the area fine. Just give the scratched area a quick spray of hydrogen peroxide, making sure the liquid reaches the skin and does not end up sitting only on the fur. Repeat over the next few days, if scratch appears to be infected.

Rid your home of cat urine odor by dousing with liberal amounts of hydrogen peroxide and allowing to rest a few minutes until the foaming action stops. Wash away and repeat, if necessary.

Dogs

Give dogs a loving bath in a solution of ¼ cup hydrogen peroxide to every gallon of warm water. You can also add a dog's favorite shampoo, if you wish. Rub and scrub through hair being sure to massage deep into fur. Rinse several times thoroughly with warm water.

Give your dog a spray bath by spraying with a hydrogen peroxide and water solution, 50/50 solution. Rub through fur and hair. Rinse with a garden hose and dry.

Has your hunting dog been sprayed by a skunk? Try this remedy. In a large bucket, mix 3 or 4 cups of hydrogen peroxide, ½ cup baking soda, 1 cup of water and a few squirts of liquid dish soap. Wash dog in solution being careful to rub the concentration deep into your pet's skin. Allow to remain on dog for 5 or 10 minutes, and then rinse thoroughly clean. Repeat if necessary.

Disinfect over clipped nails by gently spraying with peroxide.

Skunk spray

Have you or your pet been sprayed by a skunk? Get rid of the odor. In a bathtub filled half full of warm water, add 4 or 5 cups of hydrogen peroxide, 1 cup baking soda, and a few tablespoons of liquid dish soap. Wash with tub solution being careful to avoid tender areas of the skin, especially the eyes. Rinse thoroughly and repeat if necessary.

Mix a solution of hand soap and hydrogen peroxide to wash self of skunk spray odor.

MISCELLANEOUS

Contact lenses

Have your contact lenses been dropped or exposed to possible bacteria? Clean and disinfect by soaking in hydrogen peroxide for 30-40 minutes, followed by rinsing in a neutralizing solution. Contact lenses must be rinsed in the neutralizing solution prior to being used.

Taxidermy uses

Clean and whiten bones and skulls with hydrogen peroxide. For taxidermy uses, you can use 35% hydrogen peroxide grade. Remember at this strength to use gloves when handling the peroxide as it can damage skin. Clean bones or skull as best you can and place into a small plastic tub. With a paint brush, paint on hydrogen peroxide, remembering to reach all crevices. Allow to set undisturbed overnight, out of reach of children or animals. Bones should be whitened by morning. Repeat if necessary.

Serious decontamination

Hydrogen peroxide has been used for anthrax decontamination.

Waste and sewage spills

Hydrogen peroxide can be used to treat waste dump areas, ridding the dumps of dangerous and harmful bacteria. Sewage spills and dumps can also be cleaned and disinfected with hydrogen peroxide.

Purifying water

Hydrogen peroxide can be safely used to purify drinking water in case of an emergency.

Humidifiers

Add about 2 cups of hydrogen peroxide to each gallon of water in your humidifier. It is a method to deliver hydrogen peroxide gently to your respiratory system as well as keeping your humidifier clean and free of germs and bacteria.

Roof stains

Some people claim spraying hydrogen peroxide onto stained or moldy roof shingles can remove the dark stain. Spray peroxide onto the stained area and allow to stand for a couple of hours. Spray off with a garden hose. Do NOT use a power wash sprayer, as this can damage shingles.

Preserving Milk

It has been said that adding a teaspoon of food grade (35%) hydrogen peroxide to a fresh gallon jug of milk will help keep it lasting longer in your refrigerator.

Clean your fishing boat

Clean fish gunk and blood from your fishing boat by scrubbing with a concentration of food grade (35%) hydrogen peroxide and a scrub brush. Since higher grade peroxide can be extremely irritating to skin, care should be used when using by wearing protective gloves. Be careful not to splash or spray peroxide into eyes.

Swine flu

Some people believe a rigorous regimen of hydrogen peroxide will stave off the swine flu virus.

According to the CDCs website, hydrogen peroxide is useful in destroying influenza viruses, when properly used. Be sure and wash down hands and surfaces such as doorknobs and countertops for an extended period of time to destroy and hamper the spread of the virus.

Europeans of Old used hydrogen peroxide to kill bodily infections by placing drops of peroxide into the ear canal at the onset of illness. During the world-wide flu outbreak of 1918, physicians used this data as a basis for treatment for those suffering from flu, by directly injecting the patient with peroxide.

Blood stream

Scientists are researching hydrogen peroxide's benefit of introducing more oxygen into the blood stream as a way of combating major illnesses.

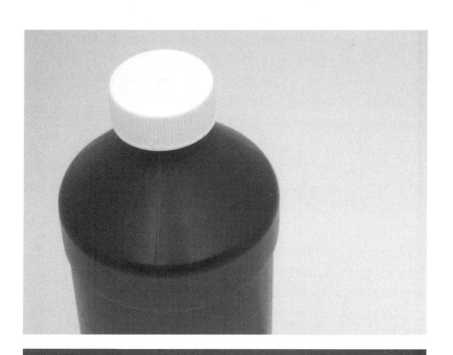

CHAPTER SIX
The Great Outdoors

Now that we have discovered a multitude of cleaning uses for hydrogen peroxide inside the home, let's head outside! Outdoors, hydrogen peroxide can be used everywhere from patios and decks to gardens and swimming pools!

Hydrogen peroxide, being an element found abundantly in nature, is a perfect companion to outdoor use. While the science of hydrogen peroxide as a component to gardening, cleaning and as an oxidizer are still being researched (and sometimes debated), science has already opened the field wide open with many useful discoveries. And, more are being discovered by readers like you each and every day:

- Germ and bacteria killer

- Plant oxidizer

- Fertilizer

- Insecticide

- Pesticide

- Disinfectant

- Antifungal spray

- Antimicrobial treatment

- Algae eliminator

This amazing liquid can be safely used outdoors without concern for hurting the environment. Plus, it's inexpensive and easy to find in stores. The uses for hydrogen peroxide are endless!

Watering Gardens – Better than Water Alone?

A little background on this subject will go a long way in explaining the potential benefits of adding hydrogen peroxide to your gardens and plant life.

Hydrogen peroxide (H_2O_2), as we have previously discussed, is simply the water molecule (H_2O_2) plus an additional oxygen atom. This "oxygenated" water is what makes hydrogen peroxide so unique, and so effective.

Why is this important?

As rain waters down on our gardens, it picks up random, floating oxygen atoms in the atmosphere along the way. As this "oxygenized" rain falls down onto plants and gardens, vegetation receives a wonderful oxygen boost, in the form of hydrogen peroxide. This boost of natural oxygen results in rich vegetation growth. This is why natural occurring rainwater produces richer plant life than watering with water from a garden hose. It gets the benefit of the extra oxygen atom that has been caught up in the raining water.

That's not to say one shouldn't water a garden with water from a garden hose. But, science is showing we may be closer to being able to replicate nature than we once thought! By adding hydrogen peroxide to our garden water, plants are receiving the identical type oxygenated watering they thrive on so beautifully with rain water.

Research is still relatively new on the benefits of using hydrogen peroxide as a gardening supplement. But, many gardeners are convinced hydrogen peroxide is the reason they have lush vegetation as well as higher volume crops season after season.

A Powerful Insecticide and Antifungal Solution
In addition to the oxygen it releases for plant growth, hydrogen peroxide is very beneficial to gardening for its insecticide and antifungal properties.

The Environmental Protection Agency has approved hydrogen peroxide as an ingredient for controlling pests and insects so destructive to farmer's crops and fields. This peroxide has been found to be beneficial in controlling or eliminating bacteria and fungus growing on plants, and also a major source of plant disease.

Hydrogen peroxide seems to work best as a pesticide when used at 1% or less. This means diluting peroxide in water before spraying it onto plants and crops.

It is recommended that spray should be used on foliage, as well as pretreating the soil or roots through saturation.

One could also assume that spraying this diluted hydrogen peroxide solution directly onto vegetables themselves would be beneficial, since we also use the liquid as a vegetable wash. As with any garden vegetable, be sure to rinse or wash before eating, to be sure dirt and soil have been removed.

Outdoor Living Areas

Outdoor living areas can be a wonderful, quiet retreat, secluded from the hustle and bustle of day to day living. But, they can rapidly be rendered unusable if mold and mildew become a problem. Sometimes the very shade that gives us a bit of refuge from harsh sunlight provides the very stage for mold and mildew to begin growing. The shady areas of our decks and patios are natural places for that mold to take hold and grow. All of a sudden, our beautiful refuge is taken over by unsightly and potentially harmful mold and mildew.

Poor draining can cause stagnant water to build up and before we know it, mildew is rampant. White plastic outdoor furniture seems to be a magnet for that dingy mildew, too.

The same traits that make hydrogen peroxide perfect for plants and gardens also make it a good fighter of mold and mildew. A few sprays or soaks quickly oxidize and break up fungus formations. Bacterial mold is killed off through oxidation.

Effective on Ponds and Pools

And what about swimming pools and ponds? -Hydrogen peroxide can help with that slippery mildew scum that builds up on the edges of ponds and pools. Fountain algae dies, as well as bacteria that can be found in stagnant water.

Environmentally Safe

Best of all, you won't have to worry about introducing harmful chemicals to the garden vegetables your family eats, or to the environment. Over just a short period of time, exposure to air and sunlight causes the breakdown of hydrogen peroxide into water and oxygen. These end-game molecules are not harmful to the environment...instead they are actually beneficial!

Worried about harming the little critters that co-inhabit your yard? Hydrogen peroxide is also safe for animals.

The following pages contain some ideas that have been proven effective in outdoor use. There are also a few ideas from people just like you. Useful ways to get the most out of a little bottle.

So, let's get started!

IN THE GARDEN

Black mold on plants

To eliminate black mold growing on plants, try mixing 1 cup of 35% hydrogen peroxide into about 6 gallons of water. Use your garden sprayer to spray down plants where black garden mold has taken hold. Repeat every day for one week.

To prevent mold or fungus from taking hold of plants, spray a weekly watering of hydrogen peroxide diluted in water directly onto plant leaves.

General gardening

Keep plants green and beautiful by gently spraying leaves with hydrogen peroxide on a weekly basis.

Prior to planting your garden, use hydrogen peroxide to prepare the soil. Soak the soil in hydrogen peroxide and water mixture and allow liquid to seep deep into soil. This will help keep bacteria, fungus and other living organisms from thriving in garden soil.

As you prepare to add delicate seedlings to garden soil, consider soaking them briefly in a hydrogen peroxide solution. The solution should be 1 part hydrogen peroxide, 3 parts water. Soak for a few minutes before introducing to the soil. Plant diseases will be kept to a minimum.

Fungicide

Get rid of garden fungus with this mixture. Combine 1 cup hydrogen peroxide and 1 gallon of water. Pour solution onto soil where fungus is a problem.

Insecticide

Mix a solution of 1 cup hydrogen peroxide and 1 gallon of water. Pour into a spray bottle and spray plants where aphids and other plant eating bugs are taking over your garden.

Many people say spraying hydrogen peroxide combined with a solution of water directly onto plant leaves will act as a natural insecticide, ridding your garden of unwanted bugs and insects.

Saturate soil around plants where insects are a problem with hydrogen peroxide.

Mix a powerful insecticide for use in the most troubled areas of your vegetable garden. Combine 3 tablespoons hydrogen peroxide, 2 tablespoons sugar and 2 cups of water in a plastic spray bottle. Use liberally on plants affected with aphids, ants or other plant eating insects.

Fertilizer

Mix a solution of hydrogen peroxide using 1 tablespoon for every gallon of water. Spray on plants and surrounding soil. This will inhibit root rot and make for stronger, healthier roots. With healthier roots, plants will grow stronger and larger.

Compost piles

Keep bacteria from compost piles from building up by dousing with hydrogen peroxide and water sprayed periodically.

Oxidizer

Simulate rainwater's healthy oxidation by adding peroxide to your garden's watering. Combine 1 part hydrogen peroxide to 3 parts water and spray liberally over garden vegetation for lush, healthy crops.

One can also use a spray attachment to add peroxide to your garden. Clean out a used, empty bottle of liquid garden fertilizer (the bottles that attach directly to a garden hose sprayer). Fill with hydrogen peroxide and attach back to your hose. Spray liberally at least once a week in your garden and on ornamental plants.

Weed killer
Some people say spraying hydrogen peroxide on unwanted weeds will cause their demise.

It has been said that 8 – 10% hydrogen peroxide will kill weeds when sprayed directly on leaves. Be careful not to spray nearby healthy and wanted plants.

Mushrooms
Use hydrogen peroxide to grow mushrooms indoors in a sterile, bacteria-free environment.

Trees
Spray on cut tree branches to prevent bacteria and infection that could damage tree.

Put an ounce or two of hydrogen peroxide into a quart of water. Spray onto tree fungus to kill the fungus without harming the tree.

Spray fruit trees with food grade (35%) hydrogen peroxide diluted in water to keep disease from harming tree.

Root rot
Prevent root rot by spraying plants and trees with hydrogen peroxide. Extra oxygen in the peroxide will help dry up root rot and allow healing to begin.

Spraying plants with peroxide will also fight over watering, as the extra oxygen atom acts to dry up over watering problems. The oxygen breaks up extra space in the roots occupied by water and waits for air to refill the holes.

Diseased plants
Spray household grade (3%) hydrogen peroxide directly onto the leaves of diseased plants once or twice a week.

Douse soil of sick or diseased plants with hydrogen peroxide diluted in water to give a quick oxygen boost. Also spray leaves and stems.

Drought
For plants that have been affected by drought, freshen with a solution of ½ cup hydrogen peroxide mixed into a gallon of water until plants return to health.

Garden flowers
Mix an ounce or two of hydrogen peroxide into 4 cups of water. Spray onto garden flowers to encourage growth.

Want longevity to cut flowers? Try adding a capful of hydrogen peroxide to vase water. This will keep bacteria from growing that could damage delicate flowers and shorten their life span.

Seedlings
Do you soak your seeds in water overnight to give them a head start? Try this for even greater growth! Combine 1 or 2 tablespoons hydrogen peroxide into 1 or 2 cups of

water. Soak seeds overnight before planting to maximize and encourage rapid growth!

For an even more vigorous start, oxidize the soil where seeds are going to be planted prior to planting. Saturate soil with a hydrogen peroxide and water mix and allow to seep into soil. Plant seeds that have been soaking overnight in peroxide solution.

Greenhouses
Spray hydrogen peroxide in greenhouses to keep down fungus or mold build up.

Pools and Ponds

Algae
Remove that slippery green algae covering pond rocks and stones. Spray with a light coating of hydrogen peroxide solution every day for 5 or 6 days to rid area of algae build up.

For thicker algae, it may be necessary to repeat for a few extra days.

Pour hydrogen peroxide into ponds to rid them of excess algae.

Coy ponds
Add a small amount of hydrogen peroxide to keep algae and slime build up from your expensive coy fish ponds. (Sometimes called Koi fish.)

Many parasitic diseases in coy fish can be treated with hydrogen peroxide blotted directly on the wound, or added to their environment.

Pour a little hydrogen peroxide into your coy fish pond to prevent bacterial and parasitic diseases from being spread.

Keeping a little peroxide sprayed around the edges of your ornamental pond will keep that slippery slime from forming. It is also good for surrounding vegetation and plant life.

Fountains

Keep outdoor fountains beautiful and algae-free by periodically dumping a cup or two of hydrogen peroxide into the fountain water. It is safe for the pumping mechanism as well as being safe for any outdoor critters that may be drinking from the fountain's water.

Spray down ornamental water fountains with hydrogen peroxide as a preventative measure to keep green algae build up at bay.

Inflatable pools

Keep a little hydrogen peroxide on hand to spray down a child's inflatable pool between uses. This will keep mold from forming and keep pool disinfected from germs.

Chlorine replacement

Many people use hydrogen peroxide to replace harsh chlorine in pools, hot tubs and even public baths.

Pool tools

Use hydrogen peroxide to keep pool tools and netting free from algae or scum.

Rust spots

Eliminate dingy rust spots with a mixture of hydrogen peroxide and baking soda. Rub mixture into rusted spot and allow to rest at least 20 minutes before scrubbing clean.

DECKS AND PATIOS

Regularly spray plastic deck furniture that is located in the shade with hydrogen peroxide to keep mold and fungus from beginning to grow.

Spray hydrogen peroxide diluted in water on patio umbrellas. If using a strong peroxide mix, be sure and test fabric umbrellas for color fastness prior to using.

Bacteria can easily accumulate on outdoor patio or deck furniture. Keep clean by having a spray bottle of hydrogen peroxide on hand to spray down and wipe table prior to eating on.

Plastic decks can be washed clean like new without the use of a power washer by spraying with hydrogen peroxide diluted in water. Spray down deck and leave on for 20 – 30 minutes. Rinse deck clean with water and allow to sun dry. Repeat, if necessary.

Barbecue Grills

Easily clean barbecue grills with a solution of hydrogen peroxide and baking soda. Remove grill grate from a barbecue grill in need of a good cleaning. Spray grate liberally with hydrogen peroxide and allow to stand for a few minutes. With a cloth or sponge dampened in peroxide and coated in baking soda, gently scrub grates clean. Rinse and dry.

For grill grates with baked on food, clean with a scrub brush soaked in baking soda and hydrogen peroxide.

Don't forget to disinfect burner and counter portion of grill to completely clean from stray bacteria.

Clean outdoor cooking tools, such as tongs and spatulas, in hydrogen peroxide regularly. This will keep bacteria from forming.

Periodically spray down bird feeder with hydrogen peroxide and wipe clean to keep mold from growing. This also helps to keep bacteria and germs from collecting.

A LITTLE MORE

Bird baths

Spray down bird baths with hydrogen peroxide, rinse with clean water and refill. This will keep algae from forming on the bird bath itself, as well as keeping bacteria at bay.

Gutters

After your fall clean up, to kill mold growing in storm gutters, pour hydrogen peroxide down gutters and wash through system with a garden hose.

Rooftops

Does your home's rooftop look dark and dingy? Much of the heavy discoloration on shingle rooftops is really mold and algae. Save money by washing the rooftop yourself with hydrogen peroxide. Using a large spray vessel, fill half full with hydrogen peroxide and half full of water. Spray down rooftop with careful attention paid to moldy areas, being sure to fully saturate the black spots. Allow to remain on rooftop for several hours before washing clean with a garden hose. Allow to dry fully in the sun. If stain is still present, continue the process again until stain is fully removed. Take caution if near the rooftop. Mold can be very slippery, and becomes more slippery when wet.

Car Deodorizer

Fill a spray bottle with a 50/50 solution of regular household strength (3%) hydrogen peroxide and water. Spray down interior car carpet and car mats with peroxide solution, and allow to air dry to remove unpleasant car odor. Hydrogen peroxide's oxidizing properties help neutralize odor naturally. Remember to always test an inconspicuous spot of carpet or fabric before use. Don't forget to spray down inside of trunk.

Wipe down any plastic, such as the dashboard or side panels, with peroxide to remove lingering odors.

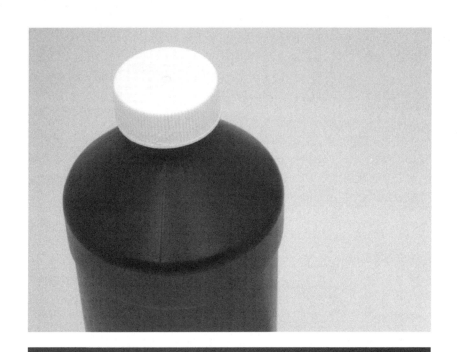

CHAPTER SEVEN
Foaming Fun

Hydrogen peroxide is used in the science world to create everything from bubbling fizz to explosive reactions. Hydrogen peroxide has been used to power cars, launch a rocket or even power a jet engine.

In science laboratories, this amazing peroxide solution is used at 30% grade as a reagent and also as a bleach in the manufacturing of paper and textiles. Slightly higher grades are used in the manufacturing of foam rubber.

It is well known that the military has used hydrogen peroxide in the highest grades of 90% - 99% as a high energy fuel for lightweight engine uses. Science continues to study uses for the explosive properties of high-grade peroxide.

The following pages contain just a few experiments you can try at home to show you firsthand the amazing power of hydrogen peroxide!

Something to keep in mind as you begin to discover the wonders of hydrogen peroxide for yourself. Hydrogen peroxide is H_2O_2. This is just the simple water molecule (H_2O) plus an extra oxygen. This extra atom of oxygen is what is responsible for many of the chemical reactions you will see taking place. That is why using straight H_2O, instead of H_2O_2 is so important!

As you are getting started, be sure and read all of the instructions carefully and use protective eye wear at all times. Gloves will be helpful in keeping your skin protected, too. Children should do the experiments in the presence of a parent or responsible adult.

Read all the instructions carefully and take precautions as necessary. Most of all, have fun discovering some of the wonderful, amazing attributes of hydrogen peroxide!

Here are a few suggestions to get you started enjoying some hydrogen peroxide fun:

1. Always use adult supervision.

2. Never drink hydrogen peroxide.

3. Make sure you are doing any "rocket" or "blast-off" experiments outdoors, away from cars, windows or pets.

4. Use safety goggles.

5. Use protective gloves to keep peroxide from irritating skin.

6. Be cautious when using hydrogen peroxide around carpet or other material you wouldn't want bleached... that includes clothing! You may wish to wear old clothes or a protective apron.

Discovering Potato Bubbles

What you need:

1 Potato

Hydrogen peroxide

Pour a little hydrogen peroxide into the palm of your hand. Unless you have an open cut or scrape, nothing should happen...no bubbling action, no fizzing. But, we all have germs on our hands, so why doesn't the hydrogen peroxide fizz??

Now take the potato and cut it in half. Pour a little hydrogen peroxide on the open part of the potato. See the bubbles and fizz??

Why does it work?

Hydrogen peroxide needs a catalyst to begin it's oxidizing, fizzing action. Even though there are germs on our hands, peroxide needs the catalyst catalase to foam. Catalase is the substance found in blood. It is also found abundantly in potatoes. That's why the fizzing action associated with hydrogen peroxide coming into contact with blood is simulated on the potato. Both contain catalase!

Heating it Up!

What you need:
½ cup 3% hydrogen peroxide
1 packet (1 tsp) dry yeast
Thermometer
Wooden stick or beverage stir stick
Small bowl

Pour hydrogen peroxide into bowl. Using your thermometer, take the temperature of the peroxide liquid and record it. Leaving the thermometer in the bowl of peroxide, add the packet of dry yeast and slowly stir with your wooden stick.

Watch the temperature change as the yeast is dissolved and bubbles begin to form and foam.

Why does it work?
The packet of yeast contains the chemical, catalase which helps release bubbles as it comes into contact with the hydrogen peroxide. The production of these bubbles causes an exothermic (heat) reaction, and raises the temperature of the bowl of peroxide.

Fizzy Fun

What you need:
Empty plastic bottle, 16 oz size
1 pkg. (I tsp) dry yeast
6% hydrogen peroxide solution
2 t. dish soap
Funnel

It is best to do this experiment outdoors, or in a bathtub where clean up is simple.

Place empty bottle on ground and put funnel into bottle neck. Pour about 4 teaspoons of hydrogen peroxide into bottle using funnel. Add the dish soap to the bottle. Quickly add the dry yeast to bottle through the funnel and remove funnel.

Watch as the bubbly foam pours out of the top of the bottle.

Why does it work?
Hydrogen peroxide is mixing with the yeast catalyst which produces the bubbling foam action.

Peroxide Breakdown

What you need:

Bottle of hydrogen peroxide (you will only use a small bit of this, not the entire bottle)

Dish or bowl

1 potato

Knife

In a small bowl, pour about a quarter cup of hydrogen peroxide. Allow to set undisturbed on the counter for several days.

In 2-3 days, carefully cut the potato in half. Pour a teaspoon of hydrogen peroxide from the dish onto the cut potato edge on one of the halves. Then pour FRESH hydrogen peroxide from the closed bottle onto a cut potato edge. Which fizzed more?

Do not discard the used hydrogen peroxide.

Keep the peroxide in the dish on the counter for another week, uncovered and undisturbed. Repeat the experiment again. Cut a potato in half and pour a teaspoon or so of the OLD hydrogen peroxide in the dish on the cut potato edge. Now pour some FRESH hydrogen peroxide onto the other cut edge of the potato. Which fizzed more?

Why does it work?

Hydrogen peroxide is the basic molecule H_2O_2, which is basic water (H_2O) plus an additional oxygen atom. Hydrogen peroxide is an unstable molecule and easily loses its extra oxygen atom, turning it into ordinary water.

Sunlight, air, age and contaminates all hasten this process. The peroxide left on the counter was subject to each of these elements, rendering it ineffective and losing its oxygen molecule as it degraded into water. The hydrogen peroxide in the bottle was kept out of damaging sunlight and away from contaminates so it held onto its oxygen molecule.

This is a great example of how and why hydrogen peroxide loses its effectiveness over time.

Blue Sky Cloud Bubbles

What you need:
Empty plastic bottle, 16 oz size
1 pkg. (I tsp) dry yeast
6% hydrogen peroxide solution
2 t. dish soap
Funnel
Blue food coloring

Place empty bottle on ground and put funnel into bottle neck. Pour about 4 teaspoons of hydrogen peroxide into bottle using funnel. Add the dish soap to the bottle, followed by a few drops of blue food coloring. Quickly add the dry yeast to bottle through the funnel and remove funnel.

Watch as blue sky cloud bubbles foam out of the bottle!

Why does it work?
Hydrogen peroxide is mixing with the yeast catalyst which produces the bubbling foam action.

Peroxide-Powered Rocket

What you need:
Empty plastic bottle, 16 oz size, with a non-screw cap
1 straw
Plastic wrap
Stick or heavy wire (needs to fit inside straw)
1 pkg. (I tsp) dry yeast
6% hydrogen peroxide solution
2 t. dish soap
Funnel

Place the thin stick or wire in the ground, a safe distance from houses, cars or people. Tape straw to outside of bottle making certain straw is level with top of bottle. Pour 1" - 2" hydrogen peroxide into bottle. Gently pour yeast in a small square of plastic wrap.

When ready to launch, wad up plastic wrap loosely (do not tie in knot…it needs to easily open) and place in bottle. Put on cap or cork, but not too tightly. Gently shake bottle to combine mixture and begin foaming action. Turn bottle upside down and place straw over stick (or wire) "launcher." Stand back and watch the launch!

Why does it work?
Hydrogen peroxide is mixing with the yeast catalyst which produces the bubbling foam action. The pressure building up inside the plastic bottle causes your rocket to launch!

Halloween Green Goop

What you need:

1 pkg. (I tsp) dry yeast

6% hydrogen peroxide solution

2 t. dish soap

Pineapple chunks or tidbits

Jack O'lantern

Green food coloring

It is best to do this experiment outdoors, or in a bathtub where clean up is simple.

Place cut jack o'lantern on ground. Pour a can of pineapple chunks or tidbits (for texture) into pumpkin along with 10 -12 drops of food coloring. Pour about 1/4 cup of hydrogen peroxide into the pumpkin. Add 2 teaspoons of dish soap. Quickly add the dry yeast to the pumpkin through the hole in the top. Replace top and watch green pumpkin goop ooze from jack o'lantern's eyes, nose and mouth.

Why does it work?

Hydrogen peroxide is mixing with the yeast catalyst which produces the bubbling foam action.

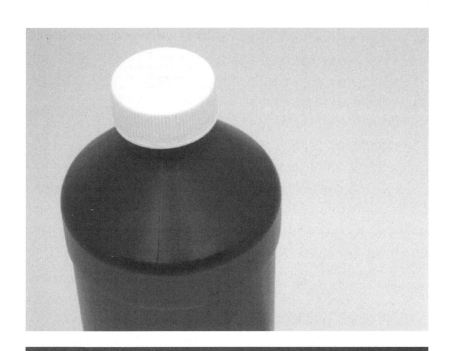

CHAPTER EIGHT

Emily Answers
Your Questions About
Hydrogen Peroxide

What should I do with my excess hydrogen peroxide?

Most excess hydrogen peroxide can be washed away down the sink drain. Particularly household grade at 3% is safe for the environment and waterways it is flushing into.

Higher grades, such as 35% that is used for taxidermy purposes and hair bleaching, can be flushed down the toilet. Dump the used peroxide into the toilet and leave for a few hours before flushing. You will be able to get one last use from the peroxide by cleaning and whitening the bowl below the waterline before flushing.

Can I ingest hydrogen peroxide?

Hydrogen peroxide should never be ingested without first consulting a health care professional.

Should I use hydrogen peroxide as an eye solution?

Even though hydrogen peroxide is one of the ingredients used in contact cleaning solution, it should never be used directly on the eye, as this can cause damage to delicate eye tissue. Peroxide is a cleaning element in contact cleaning solution, but should never be used on its own or placed directly in the eye, as it can cause series eye damage and even loss of sight.

Does hydrogen peroxide have an odor.

Hydrogen peroxide is both colorless and odorless, but it is not tasteless.

Can I mix hydrogen peroxide and chlorine bleach?
No, it is not safe to mix peroxide and bleach. The reaction that occurs when mixing the two chemicals can be dangerous and should be avoided.

However, hydrogen peroxide can be used in the PLACE of bleach for many cleaning purposes.

Can hydrogen peroxide be harmful to my health?
As with all chemical solutions, hydrogen peroxide can be harmful, or even fatal, if misused. Care should be taken to insure the solution does not come into contact with sensitive eyes. It could also be harmful if ingested in large amounts or if it comes into contact with the lungs. Consult your healthcare professional before beginning a hydrogen peroxide regimen.

What should I do if I or someone I know ingests hydrogen peroxide?
In small amounts, household grade (3%) hydrogen peroxide should not be dangerous to one's health. Larger amounts are not a good idea, outside of a physician's direction.

However, higher concentration grades can be dangerous. Seek medical attention immediately if you suspect ingestion or overdose of hydrogen peroxide. Do not administer Syrup of Ipecac or induce vomiting unless ordered by a healthcare professional or poison control agent.

You can reach the national Poison Control hotline at 1-800-222-1222. This line is open for both emergent and non-emergent poison related health care calls, 24 hours a day, 7 days a week.

What if my skin comes into contact with hydrogen peroxide?

With prolonged use or contact with higher grade hydrogen peroxide, blistering of the skin can occur. Flush contaminated skin for at least 15 minutes with cool water.

I have accidentally splashed hydrogen peroxide into my eyes. What should I do?

Immediately flush eyes with clean water for at least 15 minutes.

How long will my bottle of hydrogen peroxide last before going bad? Does hydrogen peroxide expire?

Hydrogen peroxide will not "go bad," per se, but will become less and less potent over time. Carefully check the expiration date printed on the bottle before purchasing. Although using the solution after the expiration date is not dangerous, you may not be getting its full benefit.

It has been said that roughly a year after opening a bottle, hydrogen peroxide releases its extra oxygen molecule and turns it into harmless water.

How should I store hydrogen peroxide?
Hydrogen peroxide should be stored in a dry, dark place away from humidity, and preferably in its original dark bottle. Light will hasten the peroxide's degradation, so keeping it in its familiar brown bottle will help keep out light. Humidity will also speed up the degradation process.

How can I prolong the life of my hydrogen peroxide, particularly if I have purchased it in bulk?
Hydrogen peroxide can be safely stored in your freezer to lengthen shelf-life. Be sure bottle is tightly sealed and clearly marked. Don't be alarmed if your peroxide doesn't freeze to a rock hard solid. Hydrogen peroxide's freezing point is -2 degrees Celsius.

Is there a difference between name brand hydrogen peroxide and cheaper, store brand varieties?
Don't waste your money on name brand hydrogen peroxide. The cheaper, store brand varieties will work the same.

Is hydrogen peroxide safe for my pet?
Hydrogen peroxide is just as safe for treating your dog and cat, as it is for yourself.

Is hydrogen peroxide flammable?
No, hydrogen peroxide itself is not flammable. However, due to the oxidizing process it produces, it may cause other objects to catch fire.

Where can I purchase hydrogen peroxide?

3% household grade hydrogen peroxide can be easily purchased at most grocery or drug stores. 6% peroxide is usually available at special beauty and cosmetology stores. Higher grades of hydrogen peroxide can be dangerous for personal use and should probably be avoided.

How should I properly dispose of hydrogen peroxide?

Regular household grade hydrogen peroxide (3%) is safe to pour down your kitchen sink or flush out in a toilet or drain. Higher grades of peroxide (20 – 40%) can also be safely washed down the drain as long as it is heavily diluted in water as it is being washed away. For higher grades (above 40%), it is best to plan for professional disposal. Most cities have collection centers to drop off unused chemicals, or several drop off dates throughout the year in your community.

Is hydrogen peroxide safe for sinks and drains?

Yes, hydrogen peroxide is safe for sinks, drains and plumbing fixtures. In fact, pouring left over or used peroxide down your drain will help rid plumbing of bacteria and kill odor.

Is hydrogen peroxide safe for the environment?

YES! Hydrogen peroxide is a natural element, consisting of the water molecule plus one extra oxygen atom. The liquid is fairly unstable, so as it degrades it breaks down into water and oxygen, which quickly evaporate into the environment. It has even been proven that hydrogen peroxide can be beneficial to the environment as it oxygenates plants, rivers and streams. It is even great for using in compost dumps to cut down on bacteria. This is one product where the environment BENEFITS from its disposal!

Where can I find information on hydrogen peroxide therapy?

There are several organizations nationwide devoted entirely to peroxide therapy research and treatment. You can contact a research facility that can put you in contact with a health care provider in your area that specializes in hydrogen peroxide treatment solutions.

Bio Health Center
David A. Edwards, MD, HMD
Jean Malik, AHP
615 Sierra Rose Drive, Suite 3
Reno, NV 89511
Phone: 775-828-4055
Fax: 775-828-4255

Your personal healthcare physician may also be able to provide you information about hydrogen peroxide therapy.

Emily, you have written several books on different and amazing ways to treat everyday maladies both safely

and naturally. How do I know which natural health option is best for me?

What a wonderful question! Yes, I have written several additional books on traditional, natural healing methods and remedies highlighting everything from vinegar to baking soda and now hydrogen peroxide. Many readers are unsure about which product to use in a given situation. To help you decide which product may work best for you as a home remedy or cleaning solution, try referring to the list in the Appendices section of this book. And don't forget to let me know of any new and amazing uses you discover on your own!

Now it's your turn! Do you have a question for Emily? What about a health remedy of your own to share? You can reach Emily by writing:

Emily Thacker
PO Box 980
Hartville, OH 44632
U.S.A.

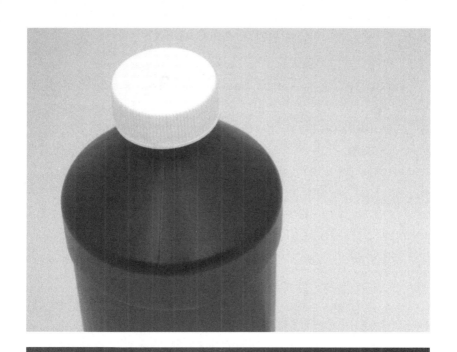

CHAPTER NINE
A Word of Caution

A NOTE OF CAUTION

While hydrogen peroxide can act as a miracle worker on tough laundry stains and whitening teeth or lightening a darkened skin spot, it is a chemical and care should be taken accordingly. There are many benefits to hydrogen peroxide's use, but with many things, prolonged use can have negative health impact. As with all home remedies, you should consult a physician before beginning any new regimen. The remedies in this book are not intended to take the place of consulting your personal healthcare physician.

As you have read, some of the ideas in this book are fact, and some are folklore. Some are suggestions and some are ideas other readers, like yourself, have tried. What may have worked for one person, may not work for your particular situation or condition.

If you have a medical problem, please consult a physician.

Keep in mind a few important reminders as you begin to make hydrogen peroxide part of your daily living:

Bleaching action
Hydrogen peroxide is a type of bleaching solution. Care should be taken when using hydrogen peroxide for the first time on fabrics and carpets to be sure peroxide will not have a negative effect on favorite fabrics. You can test hydrogen peroxide's use on a small area of fabric or carpet before treating the entire area.

Cuts and wounds

Hydrogen peroxide should never be used on deep tissue cuts and wounds, as this will hamper the healing process of delicate tissue. Peroxide can be safely used on minor cuts, scrapes and abrasions that do not run deep.

Eyes

Care should be taken to avoid getting hydrogen peroxide into sensitive eye areas.

Ingesting

Although some remedies have been known to ingest light amounts of hydrogen peroxide, this should only be done with the approval of a health care provider. In general, hydrogen peroxide should not be ingested.

Ingesting food-grade or higher concentrations of hydrogen peroxide can cause abdominal cramping, ulcers, breathing problems, seizures and even death.

Skin

As with most things, use hydrogen peroxide on your skin in moderation. Just as hydrogen peroxide works to bubble away bacteria on cuts and scrapes, it can also damage surrounding tissue after prolonged use. This can sometimes lengthen healing times which opens the door to infection. If you use hydrogen peroxide on cuts or abrasions, do so sparingly and only for short periods of time.

Inhalation

Inhaling large amounts of hydrogen peroxide, or hydrogen peroxide in higher grades, can be dangerous to the lungs, or even fatal.

Inhaling household (3%) hydrogen peroxide can cause respiratory inflammation. Inhaling hydrogen peroxide in higher grade concentrations can cause permanent lung damage or be fatal.

Flammable liquid

Hydrogen peroxide in higher grades can be flammable or even explosive. Great care, if not avoidance, should be given when handling the solution in these concentrations.

Tender membranes

Prolonged use of hydrogen peroxide on areas with tender mucous membranes, such as nostrils or mouths, should be avoided as damage could occur with repeated use.

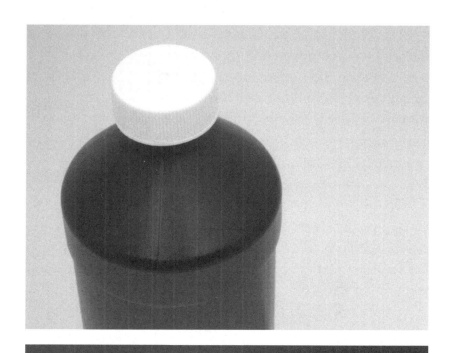

CHAPTER TEN

Appendices

This book is just one in a series of books Emily Thacker has written on old time natural ways of maintaining health and of easing the aggravation of minor everyday ills. Her books also show you how to clean up around the house and fight pests in the garden and lawn – all without using dangerous chemicals, harming the environment or using potentially harmful drugs.

Emily's books show that apple cider vinegar, baking soda, hydrogen peroxide, garlic and green tea are all useful additions to a healthy lifestyle. Each one brings its own special properties to our lives. In some situations you will probably find that hydrogen peroxide will be the best thing to reach for. At other times you may find that using vinegar, baking soda, garlic or green tea is more helpful.

For example, if you have a sore throat, you may find that a little apple cider vinegar, stirred into a glass of water, makes a very helpful gargle. It is a good choice because it kills both bacteria and viruses and because when vinegar is diluted in water it is very safe to use, even fairly frequently.

Occasionally, you may find that a little drugstore-variety hydrogen peroxide, stirred into a full glass of water, is a good germ-fighting gargle, too. But, this solution is not one you would want to use every day as it has properties that, if used too frequently, would cause harm to delicate mouth and throat tissues.

Also, you might choose to treat that same sore throat with a syrup made of garlic and honey, to help your body fight the infection of a cold or the flu. Green tea and garlic also make a healing broth for treating sore throats.

Another example of the choices you have is in treating insect bites. Because of the many different kinds of itches these bites produce, you may find several different substances that are effective in calming the itch and reducing the swelling they cause. These substances would include apple cider vinegar, baking soda, hydrogen peroxide or even a compress of wet green tea leaves! Which one works best for a particular itch may require some trial and error testing on your part.

In addition, each of our bodies and immune systems are created unique. So, it is reasonable to assume that different remedies have different success rates with different people. In your search for natural and safe home remedies, you may find that one of the substances works better on your body than another. While your best friend shared wonderful results with using baking soda, your body may react better with vinegar. Keep searching for what works best for you and don't give up.

So, "what" should I use "when?"

The charts that follow will help you to explore your options for treating everyday aches and pains and for cleaning up around the home and garden. Use it to help you choose exactly the right natural substance for each particular situation.

To find out more about any of these books, check out the publisher's website:

http://www.jamesdirect.com

or, books may be purchased using the order form at the end of this book.

HOME REMEDIES

CONDITION	VINEGAR	BAKING SODA	HYDROGEN PEROXIDE	GARLIC	GREEN TEA
Acid reflux	X	X			
Acne	X	X	X	X	X
Allergies	X				
Arthritis	X			X	X
Asthma	X			X	
Athlete's foot	X	X	X		X
Bladder infection	X	X			
Body odor	X	X	X		X
Bruises	X			X	
Burns (alkali)	X				
Burns (acid)		X			
Cholesterol	X			X	X
Colds	X		X	X	
Congestion	X			X	
Constipation	X				

HOME REMEDIES

CONDITION	VINEGAR	BAKING SODA	HYDROGEN PEROXIDE	GARLIC	GREEN TEA
Cuts	X		X		
Dandruff	X	X	X	X	X
Dehydration	X	X			X
Diaper rash	X	X			X
Diarrhea	X			X	
Ear aches/infection/wax	X		X		
Flu	X			X	
Foot fungus	X		X	X	
Foot odor	X	X	X		X
Gas	X	X			
Gout	X			X	
Halitosis (bad breath)	X	X			
Headaches	X			X	
Heartburn	X	X		X	
Hemorrhoids	X			X	

HOME REMEDIES

CONDITION	VINEGAR	BAKING SODA	HYDROGEN PEROXIDE	GARLIC	GREEN TEA
High blood pressure	X			X	
Indigestion	X	X			X
Insect bites and stings	X	X	X	X	X
Insomnia	X				X
Itchy skin	X	X			X
Memory help	X			X	X
Rashes	X	X	X		X
Sore muscles	X			X	
Sore throat	X		X	X	
Sunburn	X	X			X
Toothaches	X		X		X
Weight loss	X				X
Wound cleanser			X		
Yeast infection	X		X	X	
Youthful skin	X				

AROUND THE HOME

APPLICATION	VINEGAR	BAKING SODA	HYDROGEN PEROXIDE	GARLIC	GREEN TEA
Appliance cleaning	X	X	X		
Automobiles	X	X	X		
Bathroom fixtures	X	X	X		
Carpets, rugs, upholstery	X	X	X		
Cleaners	X	X	X		
Crafts	X	X	X	X	X
Cutting boards	X	X	X		
De-icer	X	X			
Denture soak	X		X		
Deodorizor	X	X			
Dishwasher odors	X	X	X		
Disinfecting	X	X	X		
Drains	X	X			
Fertilizer	X		X		X
Floors	X	X	X		

AROUND THE HOME

APPLICATION	VINEGAR	BAKING SODA	HYDROGEN PEROXIDE	GARLIC	GREEN TEA
Garbage disposal odors	X	X	X		
Gardening	X	X	X		X
Grease fighter	X	X	X		
Grease fires		X			
Insect control	X	X	X	X	
Jewelry cleaning	X	X	X		
Kitchen fires		X			
Laundry	X	X	X		
Mirrors	X	X	X		
Mold/mildew	X	X	X		
Odors, kitchen	X	X	X		X
Odors, feet	X	X	X		
Odors, shoes		X			
Outdoor furniture	X	X	X		
Pets	X	X	X	X	X

AROUND THE HOME

APPLICATION	VINEGAR	BAKING SODA	HYDROGEN PEROXIDE	GARLIC	GREEN TEA
Plant pests	X	X	X	X	X
Pools	X	X	X		
Pool ph control		X			
Pots and pans	X	X	X		
Showers, soap scum	X		X		
Skunk odors	X	X	X		
Smoke damage	X	X	X		
Stains, dishes	X	X	X		
Stain remover	X	X	X		
Soap extender	X	X			
Tile and grout	X	X	X		
Toilet cleaning	X	X	X		
Water softener		X			
Weed control	X	X	X		
Windows	X	X	X		

COOKING

MISCELLANEOUS	VINEGAR	BAKING SODA	HYDROGEN PEROXIDE	GARLIC	GREEN TEA
Acidic foods		X			
Baking	X	X		X	X
Bread leavening		X			
Cooking	X	X		X	X
Desserts	X	X		X	X
Dressings	X			X	X
Drinks	X			X	X
Fizzy beverages	X	X			
Herbs	X			X	X
Hunters/wild game	X	X			
Marinades	X			X	X
Meat tenderizer	X	X		X	
Pickling	X				
Sauces	X			X	X
Soups	X			X	X

List of Physicians

The following is a referral list of physicians who educate in the field of oxidative medicine. It is given with the understanding that the publisher is not engaged in rendering medical advice and does not intend this as a substitute for medical care by qualified professionals. No claims are intended as to the safety, or endorsing the effectiveness of any specific method, nor does it recommend its practice.

Arizona

Gordon Josephs, D.O.
CCUSA
C/O 7315 E. Evans Rd.
Scottsdale, AZ 85260
P 480-998-9232
F 480-998-1528

David C. Korn, D.D.S., D.O.,
   M.D. (H)
Longlife Medical, Inc.
6632 E. Baseline Rd
   Ste. 101
Mesa, AZ 85206
P 480-354-6700
F 480-354-6708

Charles D. Schwengel, D.O.
Medicine of Hope,
   Integrative Cancer
   Care
1215 E. Brown Rd. Ste. 2
Mesa, AZ 85203
P 480-668-1448

Arkansas

Melissa Taliaferro, M.D.*
P.O. Box 400
Leslie, AR 72645
P 870-447-2599
F 870-447-2917

California

Rita Ellithorpe, M.D.
Sellman Health and
   Longevity Institute
13372 Newport Ave, Suite O
Tustin, CA 92780
P 714-544-1521
F 714-544-3467

Florida

Martin Dayton, D.O.
18600 Collins Avenue
Sunny Isle Beach, FL 33160
P 305-931-8484
F 305-936-1849

Nelson Kraucek, M.D.
Life Family Practice
1501 US Hwy. 441 N.,
    Suite 1706
The Villages, FL 32139
P 352-750-4333
F 352-750-2023
chealtor@aol.com

Gary L. Pynkel, D.O.*
3840 Colonial Blvd., Ste. 1
Ft. Myers, FL 33912
P 239-278-3377
F 239-278-5266

John Monhollon, M.D.
Florida Integrative Medical
    Center
2415 University Pkwy.,
    Suite 218
Sarasota, FL 34243
P 941-955-6220
F 941-955-1410

Mike Bauerschmidt, M.D.
IV Nutrition Therapies
3079 E Commercial Blvd.,
    Suite 201
Fort Lauderdale, FL 33308
P 954-306-6497

Georgia

Robert A. Burkich, M.D.
148 Scruggs Rd.
Ringgold, GA 30736
P 706-891-1200
F 706-891-1202

Illinois

Thomas L. Hesselink, M.D.
888 S. Edgelawn Dr.
Aurora, IL 60506
P 630-844-0011
F 630-844-0500

Nevada

Robert D. Milne, M.D.
Milne Medical Center
2110 Pinto Lane
Las Vegas, NV 89106
P 702-385-1393
F 702-385-4170

New York

Richard J. Ucci, M.D.*
521 Main Street
Oneonta, NY 13820
P 607-432-8752
F 607-431-9641

North Carolina

Dennis Fera, M.D.
Holistic Health &
    Medicine
1000 Corporate Dr.,
    Ste. 209
Hillsborough, NC 27278
P 919-732-2287
F 919-732-3176
holistic-med@
    mindspring.com

Oklahoma

Richard Santelli, D.C.*
Moore Family Clinic
1227 N. Santa Fe, Suite B
Moore, OK 73160
P 405-799-4436
F 405-793-1546
rsant1050@aol.com

Michael Taylor, D.C.*
Taylor Clinic
3808 E. 51st Street
Tulsa, OK 74135
P 918-749-3797
F 918-749-1536

Robert L. White, Ph.D.*
Genesis Medical
    Research Foundation
817 SW 89th Ste. D
Oklahoma City, OK 73139
P 405-634-7855
F 405-634-0778

Oregon

Terrance Young, M.D.
Cornerstone
1205 Wallace Road NW
Salem, OR 97304
P 503-371-1558
F 503-375-3866

Pennsylvania

Roy E. Kerry, M.D.
Ear Nose Throat &
    Allergy Associates, PC
17 Sixth Ave.
Greenville, PA 16125
P 724-588-2600
F 724-588-6427

Texas

Michael E. Truman, D.O.
Holistic Wellness Center
2401 Canton Dr.
Ft. Worth, TX 76112
P 817-446-5500
F 817-446-5509

Virginia

Denise E. Bruner, M.D.
5015 Lee Highway,
    Ste. 201
Arlington, VA 22207
P 703-558-4949
F 703-558-4980

Joan M. Resk, D.O.
To Life!
5303 Clearbrook Village
    Lane
Roanoke, VA 24014
P 540-776-8331
F 540-776-8303

THE VINEGAR ANNIVERSARY BOOK

THE VINEGAR ANNIVERSARY BOOK blends the contents of Emily Thacker's four books on vinegar into one big book! Plus it includes the newest research and very latest home remedies.

The original *VINEGAR BOOK* details hundreds of old time healing remedies plus information on how to clean with vinegar. You will learn about the many different kinds of vinegar – from apple cider, wine, rice and malt to more exotic kinds such as banana and date.

THE VINEGAR BOOK II offers 365 vinegar uses to let you try a new one every day of the year.

THE VINEGAR HOME GUIDE focuses on using vinegar for cleaning and disinfecting around the home, yard and garden.

THE VINEGAR DIET BOOK brings all the healthy goodness of vinegar to the table in an exciting, safe way to easily control weight. This remarkable way to manage weight offers wholesome, nourishing insight into managing what you eat. You will find this is the easiest, most foolproof diet plan you have ever tried!

To find out more about *THE VINEGAR ANNIVERSARY BOOK*, see the publisher's website: http://www.jamesdirect.com or buy it using the order form at the end of this book.

Excerpts from
THE VINEGAR ANNIVERSARY BOOK

"Vinegar is part of a healthy diet and has been used for centuries to aid health. Scientists tell us vinegar was probably part of the primordial soup of life. It is needed to burn fats and carbohydrates. The acid we know as vinegar is also used by the body as an aid in neutralizing poisons."

"Fortified vinegars contain fruits and vegetables, blended with vinegar, to form toppings and sauces. Recipes for several diet fortifying vinegars can be found in this book."

"Banish foot odor by soaking feet in strong tea. Follow with a rinse made from a cup of warm water and a cup of apple cider vinegar."

"Old times have long recommended taking a teaspoon of apple cider vinegar, every day, in a tall glass of water."

"As little as one tablespoon of vinegar per quart of water can make a difference in the calcium that is pulled from boiled soup bones."

"Vinegar, added to fish dishes, helps to eliminate the traditional fishy odor. It also helps get rid of fish smells at clean up time."

"Soak fresh vegetables in water with a little vinegar added to it to rid them of garden bugs."

Index

Acne: 88, 93 - 94
Age spots: 92
Algae: 118, 129, 135 - 139
Allergies: 76, 80
Alzheimer's: 21 - 22, 29, 80
Animal bites: 40, 74
Arthritis: 69
Asthma: 76, 80
Athletes foot: 68 - 69, 72
Babies: 66, 115
Bacteria: 25, 30, 32, 34, 39, 42, 59, 61 - 66, 69, 72 - 73, 75, 88, 93, 96,
        101 - 107, 111, 116, 119, 121 - 122, 128 - 129, 131 - 134, 136 -
        138, 158, 163, 166
Bathroom: 99, 101, 111 - 113
Beauty: 24, 33, 86 - 92, 158
Bedsores: 41, 73 - 74
Bleaching agent: 7, 13, 15, 76, 86, 87, 99, 100
Blisters: 40, 69
Boils: 69, 73
Botulism: 64 - 65
Bronchitis: 43, 45, 80
Cancer: 22, 26, 28, 30, 46, 78, 80, 82, 177
Cardiovascular disease: 43, 71, 80
Cautions: 24 - 26, 40, 66, 87 - 88, 100 - 101, 117, 162 - 164
Clogged arteries: 71
Colds: 75
Cuts: 7, 14, 23, 25, 32, 41, 58, 66, 118, 163
Diabetes: 78, 80
Diapers: 115
Digestion: 65, 80
Disinfect, disinfecting: 15, 25, 34, 40, 59 - 60, 63, 65 - 66, 74, 96 - 99,
        101 - 104, 107 - 112, 114, 117 - 119, 121, 138
Ears: 66 - 68, 118
E. coli: 34, 106
Emphysema: 43, 79, 80, 81, 82
Experiments: 142 - 151
Feet: 68 - 69, 71 - 72
Fibromyalsia: 69 - 70, 80
Flu: 80, 124, 167

Fungus: 31, 39, 68 - 69, 71 - 72, 99, 101 - 102, 111 - 112, 128, - 131, 133,
    135, 137
Germs: 30, 43, 45, 61 - 66, 69, 74, 88, 99, 105 - 107, 116, 122 - 123, 136,
    138
Gingivitis: 63, 80
Hair: 15, 24, 33, 34, 50, 86, 87, 88, 90, 91, 92, 121, 154
Headaches: 61, 80
Herpes: 42, 80
HIV: 22, 26, 43, 80
Infections: 25, 30, 43, 66, 67, 69, 72, 73, 74, 75, 79, 80, 118, 133, 163, 167
Influenza (flu): 42, 80, 124, 167
Insect bites & stings: 41, 74, 80, 167
Kitchen: 34, 98, 101 - 107, 109, 114, 158
Laundry: 15, 97, 113, 114 - 115, 162
Liver: 9, 40, 42, 80
Living areas: 98, 108, 129
Mouth: 24, 27, 43 - 45, 63 - 66, 87
Mouth sores: 64
Mouthwash: 43 - 44, 61 - 62
Muscle aches: 72
Nail problems: 71, 94
Odors: 65 - 66, 108, 139
Oxygen therapy: 26 - 27, 77 - 84
Parasites: 80, 119
Parkinson's disease: 21, 29, 43, 78, 80
Pets: 100, 110, 118
Plants: 38 - 39, 99, 100, 127 - 134, 159
Rashes: 67
Rheumatism: 69 - 70
Salmonella: 104, 107
Sanitize: 8, 24, 103, 107
Shingles: 43, 80, 123
Sinus: 75, 80
Skin: 15, 23, 25 - 26, 33 - 35, 40, 44, 54 - 55, 73, 86 - 88, 90, 92 - 94,
    100, 119 - 121 - 122, 142, 156, 162 - 163
Sore throats: 41, 75 - 76, 167
Stains: 26, 63, 88, 100, 103, 105, 109 - 110, 113 - 115, 117, 123, 162
Teeth, tooth: 44, 62 - 64, 89 - 90
Tumors: 22
Ulcers: 45, 163
Yeast infections: 75

A Thank You Note
from Emily!

Thank you, once again, dear reader, for your continued interest in natural healing ways. It has been a pleasure to bring you this book, and all its exciting uses for hydrogen peroxide.

If you have a natural healing remedy, unique or special cleaning method or fun, old-time recipe that your family has used, would you consider sharing it with other readers just like yourself? If I use it in one of my upcoming books, you will receive a free copy of the book upon printing.

Please fill out the form that follow and mail it back to me. If the form is missing or isn't available, feel free to use a sheet of paper and mail your ideas in to us.

Thank you again, and my warmest wishes for a long, healthy, happy life.

Emily Thacker

Emily, here is one of my favorite uses for hydrogen peroxide:

_____

_____

_____

_____

_____

_____

Can we use your name and city when crediting this remedy in the book?

❑ Yes, please credit this remedy to:

_____

_____

_____

❑ No, please use my remedy, but do not use my name in the book.

Either way, yes or no, if I use your remedy, I'll send you a free copy of the new edition of home remedies.

Your remedy can be one which uses hydrogen peroxide, or simply one that you feel others would like to know about.

My favorite chapter in "*The Magic of Hydrogen Peroxide*" is:

_____

_____

The most helpful remedy I appreciated in "*The Magic of Hydrogen Peroxide*" is:

_____

_____

_____

_____

_____

_____

What I liked best about "*The Magic of Hydrogen Peroxide*" is:

_____

_____

_____

_____

_____

_____

_____

Would you be interested in hearing about my new cookbook when it becomes available?

_____

_____

_____

My name and mailing address is:

_____

_____

_____

_____

If you have any comments or experiences to add to the information you've read in this collection, or if you have information for subsequent editions, please address your letters to:

Emily Thacker
PO Box 980
Hartville, OH 44632

✂ please cut here

Use this coupon to order "The Magic of Hydrogen Peroxide" for a friend or family member -- or copy the ordering information onto a plain piece of paper and mail to:

The Magic of Hydrogen Peroxide
Dept. HP521
PO Box 980
Hartville, Ohio 44632

Preferred Customer Reorder Form

Order this...	If you want a book on...	Cost...	Number of Copies...
The Vinegar Anniversary Book	Completely updated with the latest research and brand new remedies and uses for apple cider vinegar. Handsome coffee table collector's edition you'll be proud to display.	$9.95	
The Magic of Baking Soda	*Plain Old Baking Soda A Drugstore in A Box?* Doctors & researchers have discovered baking soda has amazing healing properties! Over 600 health & Household Hints. *Great Recipes Too!*	$9.95	
Amish Gardening Secrets	You too can learn the special gardening secrets the Amish use to produce huge tomato plants and bountiful harvests. Information packed 800-plus collection for you to tinker with and enjoy.	$9.95	
The Vinegar Home Guide	Learn how to clean and freshen with natural, environmentally-safe vinegar in the house, garden and laundry. Plus, delicious home-style recipes!	$9.95	
Garlic: Nature's Natural Companion	Exciting scientific research on garlic's ability to promote good health. Find out for yourself why garlic has the reputation of being able to heal almost magically! Newest in Emily's series of natural heath books!	$9.95	

Any combination of the above $9.95 items qualifies for the following discounts...

Total NUMBER of $9.95 items

Order any 2 items for: $15.95	**Order any 4 items for:** $24.95
Order any 3 items for: $19.95	**Order any 5 items for:** $29.95

Order any 6 items for: $34.95 and receive 7th item FREE

Any additional items for: $5 each

FEATURED SELECTIONS

Total COST of $9.95 items

The Magic of Hydrogen Peroxide	An Ounce of Hydrogen Peroxide is worth a Pound of Cure! Hundreds of health cures, household uses & home remedy uses for hydrogen peroxide contained in this breakthrough volume.	$19.95
Hydrogen Peroxide Formula Guide	FINALLY...No more guesswork! Step-by-step instructions and specific measurements for hundreds of amazing hydrogen peroxide uses. Learn how to use hydrogen peroxide to clean your home, balance pH soil levels, use as a home remedy or beautify your life! It is all here!	$19.95
Vinegar Formula Guide	This one-of-a-kind, ground breaking book gives you exact formulas and measurements for ALL of your vinegar applications! In it you'll find step-by-step, easy-to-use instructions for home health remedies, cleaning projects and more!	$19.95
The Cinnamon Book	Research studies have found this amazing spice is loaded with health benefits. Find out how cinnamon can be used in treating common (and not so common) conditions such as diabetes, obesity, arthritis, high cholesterol and a host of other ailments.	$19.95

Order any 2 or more Featured Selections for only $10 each...

Postage & Handling	$3.98*
TOTAL	

*** Shipping of 10 or more books = $6.96**

90-DAY MONEY-BACK GUARANTEE

Please rush me the items marked above. I understand that I must be completely satisfied or I can return any item within 90 days for a full and prompt refund of my purchase price.

I am enclosing $_____ by: ❑ Check ❑ Money Order (Make checks payable to James Direct Inc)

Charge my credit card Signature _____

Card No. _____ Exp. Date _____

Name _____ Address _____

City _____ State_____ Zip _____

Telephone Number (_____) _____

❑ Yes! I'd like to know about freebies, specials and new products before they are nationally advertised. My email address is: _____

Mail To: **James Direct Inc.** • PO Box 980, Dept. A1397 • Hartville, Ohio 44632
Customer Service (330) 877-0800 • *http://www.jamesdirect.com*

THE VINEGAR ANNIVERSARY BOOK
Handsome coffee table edition and brand new information on Mother Nature's Secret Weapon – apple cider vinegar!

- -

THE MAGIC OF BAKING SODA
We all know baking soda works like magic around the house. It cleans, deodorizes & works wonders in the kitchen and in the garden. But did you know it's an effective remedy for allergies, bladder infection, heart disorders... *and MORE!*

- -

AMISH GARDENING SECRETS
There's something for everyone in *Amish Gardening Secrets.* This BIG collection contains over 800 gardening hints, suggestions, time savers and tonics that have been passed down over the years in Amish communities and elsewhere.

- -

THE VINEGAR HOME GUIDE
Emily Thacker presents her second volume of hundreds of all-new vinegar tips. Use versatile vinegar to add a low-sodium zap of flavor to your cooking, as well as getting your house "white-glove" clean for just pennies. Plus, safe and easy tips on shining and polishing brass, copper & pewter and removing stubborn stains & static cling in your laundry!

- -

GARLIC: NATURE'S NATURAL COMPANION
Explore the very latest studies and new remedies using garlic to help with cholesterol, blood pressure, asthma, arthritis, digestive disorders, bacteria, cold and flu symptoms, and MUCH MORE! Amazing cancer studies!

- -

THE MAGIC OF HYDROGEN PEROXIDE
Hundreds of health cures & home remedy uses for hydrogen peroxide. You'll be amazed to see how a little hydrogen peroxide mixed with a pinch of this or that from your cupboard can do everything from relieving chronic pain to making age spots go away! Easy household cleaning formulas too!

- -

HYDROGEN PEROXIDE FORMULA GUIDE
This unique book lists hundreds of home remedy, gardening and cleaning uses for peroxide along with exact measurements and instructions for each use. No mistakes and no guesswork.

- -

VINEGAR FORMULA GUIDE
Studies have shown vinegar to be effective at not only cleaning and disinfecting, but also as a natural home remedy for conditions such as lowering cholesterol, fighting disease, easing arthritis, improving circulation and more! Now learn the exact formulas and measurements for EACH home remedy and cleaning project in a concise, easy-to-read format! No more guesswork!

- -

THE CINNAMON BOOK
Cinnamon is rich in natural healing properties such as being an anti-oxidant, anti-inflammatory, anti-coagulant, anti-microbial, anti-parasitic, anti-tumor – just to name a few. Find out how cinnamon can be used to fight everything from simple cuts and scrapes to chronic health condition, safely and naturally!

* Each Book has its own FREE Bonus!

> All these important books carry our NO-RISK GUARANTEE. Enjoy them for three full months. If you are not 100% satisfied simply return the book(s), for a prompt, "no questions asked" refund!